The Power to Heal

THE POWER TO HEAL

Civil Rights, Medicare,
and the Struggle to Transform
America's Health Care System

DAVID BARTON SMITH

Vanderbilt University Press
Nashville

© 2016 by Vanderbilt University Press
Nashville, Tennessee 37235
All rights reserved
First printing 2016

This book is printed on acid-free paper.
Manufactured in the United States of America

This book is a recipient of the Norman L. and Roselea J.
Goldberg Prize for the best project in the area of medicine.

Library of Congress Cataloging-in-Publication Data on file

LC control number   2015042860
LC classification number LCC RA412.4
Dewey class number   368.4/200973—dc23

ISBN 978-0-8265-2106-4   (hardcover)
ISBN 978-0-8265-2107-1   (paperback)
ISBN 978-0-8265-2108-8   (ebook)

To those who awoke

to a common dream

and all who now struggle

to realize it.

Contents

Preface

Medicare is a vibrant half century old. None now attacking the Afford-able Care Act's more conservative approach to expanding access to health insurance dare voice similar objections to this far more ambi-tious and popular one. It's an anachronism. How did it happen?

Much of the story has disappeared. Medicare's birth emerged from the last turbulent stages of the civil rights era. Indeed, as the story in this book documents, it was the concealed gift of that struggle and one of its most significant accomplishments. The civil rights movement reached its full power as a transformational force with Medicare's pas-sage and implementation. The most common responses to racial and economic disparities in opportunities in our nation's history have been: "it's just the way things are" or "it just takes time." However, for the civil rights activists involved in the implementation of the Medicare program in 1966, the response was, "Now!" In four months they trans-formed the nation's hospitals from our most racially and economi-cally segregated institutions to our most integrated. In four years they changed patterns of use of health services that had persisted for half a century. The fundamental moral imperative—that those needing medi-cal care should receive it—began for the first time to reflect actual use of services. A profound transformation, now taken for granted, hap-pened almost overnight.

That victory and the ideas and heroes that made it possible deserve celebration. Their neglected gift offers hope. In no other area of Ameri-can society, still traumatized by a brutal racial history, has the dream of a racial and economic justice come as close to being realized.

The story of that transformation has been lost. At the time, fed-eral officials, politicians, and hospitals kept quiet, fearing a backlash. Most, later embarrassed about this past, had no interest in preserving the story. It just didn't fit any of the more self-serving narratives about race, health care, politics, the role of government and the private sector in the United States. Its lost heroes play no role in any of those more accepted narratives. At its heart was an odd, implausible collection of people thrown together for a few months that changed health care in the United States. Few believed what they actually accomplished was possible. I've distilled the essential pieces of the story into the six chapters of this book. In essence, we possess a too long neglected gift that offers the power to heal, and, perhaps more than ever before, we need to use it.

Pulling this story together has taken, on and off, fifty years and the help of hundreds. I am indebted to all who provided inspiration, encouragement, and clues. The participation of my two siblings, Woollcott and Barbara, and my mother, Nancy, as civil rights activists during the period described in this book first made me aware of how much of the important parts of the story had been lost.[1] I entered the health services research doctoral program at the University of Michigan in medical care organization in the fall of 1965, during the same time that Medicare was being implemented.[2] My dissertation involved fieldwork in an early HMO set up by the United Auto Workers in Detroit during the riots of 1967.[3]

It was, however, more than twenty years later that my health services research interests overlapped with that earlier personal history. I was asked to look at numbers related to disparities in black access to nursing homes in Pennsylvania in 1989 by Ann Torregrossa, Mike Campbell, and Philip Tannenbaum of the Pennsylvania Health Law Project. The conclusions triggered a class action lawsuit against the Pennsylvania secretary of welfare by the Pennsylvanian Health Law Project and led later to a similar lawsuit against the secretary of health and human services (HHS) instigated by Gordon Bonnyman of the Tennessee Justice Center and others connected to the Poverty and Race Research Action Council (PRRAC).[4] Neither was successful in gaining legal remedies, but I learned much about how the "system" worked that I could not have learned in any other way. It stimulated the submission of an application for a Robert Wood Johnson Foundation Health Policy Research Investigator Award. That award in 1994 led to a book, *Health Care Divided* (Smith 1999).[5] It was a story, as I discovered from many of the remarkable people I interviewed, most now deceased, that needed to be told more fully than was possible at the time.

Many others have since helped immeasurably in doing this. Karen

Thomas's book *Deluxe Jim Crow* helped flesh out the painful ambiguity of choices during the Jim Crow era's influx of federal funding for hospital construction initiated with the Hill-Burton Act of 1946 (Thomas 2011). John Dittmer helped describe the peculiarly central role played by a small group of activists that formed the Medical Committee for Human Rights in *The Good Doctors* (Dittmer 2009). Beatrix Hoffman's *Health Care for Some* placed it the larger history of rationing of care in the United States (Hoffman 2012). T. R. Reid in *The Healing of America* did a marvelous job of providing a readable way of placing the American health care system's peculiarities in an international context (Reid 2010). One would have to include more hopeful books on race, such as Isabel Wilkerson's *The Warmth of Other Suns*, about the impact of the Great Migration, and more pessimistic ones, such as Michelle Alexander's *The New Jim Crow*, about the growth in incarceration (Wilkerson 2010; Alexander 2012). There have also been many moving recent biographies and histories of the broader civil rights struggle. All these accounts helped inspire me to take a shot at telling the still-untold parts of the story.

The immediate stimulation to undertake such a writing project came from the interest of Barbara Berney in converting the story into a documentary film.[6] We have shared resources, and some of the documentation and interviews she and her team have tracked down have found their way into these pages. More recent papers, enriched from the insights and interaction with many colleagues, have also helped in fleshing out the story presented here.[7]

I am also indebted to those who helped in transforming crude early drafts into a more polished final product. Among these, Joan Apt, my wife and much-loved all-purpose personal critic, and Bob Uris, longtime friend, writing critic, and aging squash partner, read all parts of the manuscript and helped in many ways in making it clearer and more readable. Michael Ames, director of Vanderbilt University Press, provided much encouragement and gentle guidance. Joell Smith-Borne, managing editor, and Kathleen Kageff, who did the wonderfully clear, careful copyediting of the manuscript, helped immeasurably in transforming it into its final form as a book.

Finally, I am indebted to the inspiration of all those who played a part in providing the gift that this book is about and those who now use that gift to realize the promise it still offers for transforming America's health system.

The Power to Heal

1

Formative Years

The patterns of medical practice and its financing in the United States developed between 1894 and 1954. Scientific advances, interest group clashes over power, and underlying social attitudes about race and class shaped its development. Just as early childhood experiences shape a person, so these early years shaped most of what continues to be distinctive about the American health care system.

During this period other industrialized nations, faced with the same rapid improvements in medicine, explored ways to best distribute its benefits. The historical narrative of these other nations said, in essence, "for all our differences we have a common identity, and, just as in any functional family, we look after each other." The universal health insurance systems created in every other wealthy industrialized country became a way of expressing that common bond, the fundamental moral conclusion that no one should be denied needed medical care (see Reid 2010: 237–39).

That never happened in the United States (Hoffman 2012). Indeed, in terms of a national health care system, the United States produced the lone, stunted outlier. Its health care costs tower over other industrialized nations—more than twice the median per capita cost and twice the percentage of its gross domestic product are allocated to health care. Yet it has fewer physicians and hospital beds per capita, and its citizens receive fewer services (Squires 2011). The United States does poorly in comparison to other nations on most measures of health. For example, it ranks twenty-seventh out of thirty-four developed nations in life expectancy at birth (OECD 2014). About 16 percent of our citizens remain uninsured, and at least a similar percentage are underinsured, making any major medical expenses unaffordable (Majerol, Newkirk, and Garfield 2014, 4). As a result, people still go untreated and die, despite all the well-meaning patchwork arrangements worked out, because they can't afford the care they need. Other industrialized nations don't allow this to happen. What made the United States different?

The explanation offered by many and supported by some persuasive statistical evidence is that the US health system was, in essence, the "child" of the national equivalent of an abusive, dysfunctional family.[1] Its formative period of development, between 1896 and 1954, corresponded to the Jim Crow era—between the assertion of the legality of segregation (*Plessy v. Ferguson*, 163 US 537 [1896]) and the assertion that separate could never be equal (*Brown v. Board of Education of Topeka*, 347 US 483 [1954]). That contradiction was first brought to public attention in Gunnar Myrdal's influential book *The American Dilemma: The Negro Problem and American Democracy* (Myrdal 1944). Indeed, the book was cited in the Brown decision. Myrdal was optimistic, arguing that the American creed of democracy and fairness would, in the long run, win out over segregation and racism. Yet so much of the structure of all aspects of life in this nation was shaped in those formative years. In no area was this truer than in the structure of America's health system. Those formative years produced all the peculiar characteristics of the nation's health system and the ideological justification for these peculiarities. Just as with the child raised in an abusive dysfunctional family, it's hard to undo the destructive effects of such a formative experience. This book tells of the struggle to do just that. That struggle was a national one and not one limited to the boundaries of the Jim Crow South. The forms it would take in the North would be different but the outcomes much the same. I have chosen to focus on Chicago to illustrate this throughout the remainder of the book, but most other northern cities could have served this purpose just as well.

Race, indeed, has always been a concealed part of the logic of "American exceptionalism." Simply creating anti-discriminatory laws or regulations or professing good intentions doesn't change this. Race, and the logic of white supremacy, is hidden in the compromise patchwork solutions, the expansion of private insurance, the creation of producer cooperative solutions in the form of voluntary Blue Cross plans, the creation of the dominant voluntary hospital sector, the ideology of individualism, the opposition to public solutions, and the promotion of freedom of choice and free market solutions that have dominated, and continue to dominate, health care in the United States. All these policy choices have a disparate impact on blacks and other disadvantaged minority groups. The notion of "social solidarity," invoked in other countries, never came up as an argument for universal protections in the United States. Only during the civil rights convulsions of the 1960s did the notion of "being all in it together" have any salience. Medicare, in its essence, was the gift of the civil rights struggle. Yet the patterns of thinking developed in those earlier formative years persist, most recently in the resistance to the implementation of Obama's Affordable Care Act.

The methods of imposing racial segregation during the first half of the twentieth century differed in the North and South, but the underlying assumptions were the same. In the South, Jim Crow laws drew visible color lines reflecting the rigid caste system created during slavery. In the North, laws and customs created more invisible but just as effective color lines around black ghettos, insulating whites from the great wave of black migration to northern urban centers from the South during this period. In both, violence defended the color lines when other means failed. The degree of segregation in northern cities, such as Chicago, was equal to that of anywhere in the South. Thus, from the failure to address the aftermath of slavery, a regionally intertwined caste system emerged in the United States. That caste system was, in turn, reflected in the early organization and financing of its health system. Those who grew up or began their medical careers before the 1960s have vivid memories of how it all worked. There was nothing functional about it. Many spent the rest of their lives fighting to change it.

The Jim Crow South

The images of the Jim Crow South still shock. The abject poverty of rural blacks in the Deep South matched any in the underdeveloped world. Many still inhabited the antebellum slave shacks and were increasingly unemployed as a result of the growing mechanization of cotton farming. They lacked access to clean water, basic sanitation, and adequate nutrition, to say nothing of medical care. As a result, when in 1966 a federally supported Office of Economic Opportunity health center was finally set up in the Mississippi delta it proceeded to violate all the conventional boundaries of medical practice.

> In the absence of any other resources, whenever we saw a child
> suffering this combination of infection and malnutrition, we wrote

prescriptions for food. . . . Not just for the sick child, but for all the children in the family, because we understood that no mother was going to feed one child while the rest of her children went hungry. And we gave these prescriptions, these food orders to the people that needed them, and worked out a system under which they could go to the black grocery stores in any of the 10 towns in our service area and the grocery store would fill the prescription for food and send the bill to our health center. We paid those bills from the health center's pharmacy budget.

The state of Mississippi found out about this and concluded that, clearly, Soviet communism had arrived in the Delta. They complained to our funder in the federal government, the Office of Economic Opportunity (OEO), the War on Poverty. And OEO officials came down to see us—so upset that they were practically babbling, steam coming out of their ears, saying, "What in God's name did we think we were doing?" We said, "What's the matter?" They said, "Well, you can't give away food and charge it to the pharmacy at the health center." We said, "Why not?" They said, "Because the pharmacy at the health center is for drugs for the treatment of disease." And we said, "Well, the last time we looked in the book, the specific therapy for malnutrition was food." (Geiger 2005, 7)[2]

In the small towns, the end of paved roads and lack of street lights marked the "colored" sections, even without the pervasive signs separating whites and blacks. Larger, more affluent towns included a separate business district with the full complement of stores and services—pharmacies, medical and legal offices, and even hospitals. Perhaps most important, these neighborhoods included a growing black middle class, increasingly impatient with the existing order.

Success, in spite of the restrictions of Jim Crow, however, produced white resentment and sometimes violent retaliation.

My father's family came from Georgia, where they owned a farm. The story goes that in the 1920's, a neighboring white plantation owner wanted the land, but my granddad refused to sell it. I guess the plantation owner got angry, and the Klan came the next night, grabbed two of my grandmother's brothers and lynched them. My grandfather returned, killed the plantation owner, and escaped. My grand mom and her kids had to also escape to avoid retaliation. They ended up in Greenville, South Carolina, and my grand mom took in washing. She never saw her husband again, but they never caught him either. He ended up in the Winston-Salem area living under an assumed name. Every once in a while, she'd get word passed along about him. There was an underground thing, an understanding that you helped other blacks who got in trouble. That's how my grandmother was able to move. (qtd. in Smith 1999, 9–10)

Perhaps, in essence, the Underground Railroad didn't disappear after emancipation. A modified version of it at the beginning of the twentieth century facilitated the Great Migration. Black newspapers in Chicago and other northern cities provided the travel guides, and Pullman porters on routes to Chicago and other northern cities from the South served as its conductors. Most of the lynching and other violence that propelled the exodus stemmed from growing tensions in competing for a living rather than mob retribution for sexual offenses against white women (Olzak and Shanahan 2003; Olzak 1992). Altogether twelve hundred blacks were lynched at the hands of whites in the South between 1882 and 1930, ranging from gruesome mass public spectacles to secret executions at the hands of a few whose motives were left a mystery (Stovel 2001, 844).

The organization of health services reflected all the divisions of the caste system. In the rural areas and small towns white hospitals either excluded blacks altogether or relegated them to a few beds in a colored ward. Only in the larger, more prosperous cities did the peculiar nature of the system bear all its strange fruit—hospitals for the indigent, for private pay black patients, for private pay whites, and for Catholic and Protestant sects, all erected in the center of town a few blocks from each other for the convenience of physicians whose practices crossed the boundaries of race, class, and religion. Typically black physicians were excluded from providing care for their patients at most of these hospitals, with the possible exception of the black hospital and colored ward of the county or city hospitals serving the indigent.

Jim Crow rules forced daily rituals of public degradation whether receiving or providing medical care, shopping, or traveling. A neurosurgeon in Greensboro, North Carolina, growing up in an insulated, privileged white world, recalled his first exposure to it. "The best friend

I had growing up was a black individual. We did everything together. Just after I turned 16 and could drive we went duck hunting along the North Carolina coast. I could not take him into any restaurant. We couldn't sleep in any lodges and I had to carry food out to him and we slept in the car. It had never hit me before. I became inflamed. I didn't understand it. It wasn't fair."[3]

Some southern communities lacked any of the civility that made such youthful friendships possible. In the 1930s, police in Fort Lauderdale, Florida, tried to keep blacks out of its downtown. They arrested and used them as convict labor if they couldn't pay stiff fines for loitering. White youths in Fort Lauderdale served as vigilante enforcers. In 1937, a young black man was shot in the abdomen by a gang of white youth intent on enforcing this ban. The two hospitals in Fort Lauderdale refused to admit him, and he died before he could be transported to one of the only black hospitals in South Florida in Miami (Oliver 1985).

The incident galvanized the black community and led to the creation of a thirty-five-bed cottage hospital in Fort Lauderdale. As many as five hundred such black hospitals were created during this formative era, in response to similar exclusions (Wesley 2010). About three-quarters of these facilities were in the South. While many white hospitals provided limited accommodation to black patients in a separate "colored ward," black physicians were typically excluded. Their needs for a workshop helped stimulate the creation of many of these facilities, some privately owned by the doctors themselves. Black hospitals also served as the only places where black nurses could be trained and black physicians could receive postgraduate internship and residency experiences. In spite of these self-help efforts, finding a close-by hospital that would admit a critically injured black patient added to the risks blacks faced in traveling in the South.

Charles Drew's death became a potent symbol of the problem of hospital segregation in the South.[4] A black physician and researcher, he had done pioneer work in storing and transporting blood plasma for shipment to British troops in the early stages of World War II. The American Red Cross in 1941, in spite of the war, chose to refuse black donors. After protests, it agreed to collect blood from blacks but only on a segregated basis. That blood donations of the person whose work had contributed to supplying plasma to save the lives of soldiers fighting Nazi Germany would be subjected to such discrimination made

Drew the symbol of a national protest against the Red Cross's policies. Drew's subsequent career in medicine was similarly restricted. He became chairman of surgery at Howard University's School of Medicine and Freedman's Hospital (the oldest black hospital, established in 1862, and the only surviving remnant of federal Reconstruction efforts after the Civil War). Because of his race, Drew could not join the local chapter of the American Medical Association and thus be eligible for privileges at any of the other hospitals in the Washington, DC, area.

On the night of April 1, 1950, Drew drove with three colleagues from Washington, DC, en route to a black medical conference in Tuskegee, Alabama. Charles Watts, a student of Drew's at Howard, had driven ahead to find accommodations in Atlanta for the following night. "During those times it was not easy to find places for black people [to spend the night]. We were going to stay at the Y in Atlanta" (qtd. in Love 1996, 15). At 7:30 a.m., near the rural community of Pleasant Grove, North Carolina, Drew dozed off at the wheel, and the car swerved off the road at high speed, fatally injuring him. He was brought by ambulance to Alamance General Hospital, a forty-eight-bed facility five miles away. The county's three black doctors were excluded from privileges, and only five of its forty-eight beds were allocated to blacks in a basement ward. Drew expired, less than an hour later, in spite of the best efforts of the white medical staff, who had learned who he was. High school and undergraduate classmate and colleague Montague Cobb served as a pallbearer at the funeral and as the key leader in the national struggle to desegregate hospitals that soon followed.

The myth, widely circulated after Drew's death, was that because of his race he was denied treatment and a transfusion that could have saved his life. It was a powerful parable, not true in Drew's case, but true in others. Indeed, eight months after Drew's death, Maltheus Avery, a veteran and North Carolina A&T College student in Greensboro, had an accident in the same location and was transported to the same hospital. He was then transferred to Duke University Hospital in Durham, where its neurosurgeons could treat him for his head trauma and stop the swelling that would be fatal. Duke, however, had only fifteen beds available on their colored ward, and they were all, apparently, full. Avery was, as a consequence, transferred to Lincoln, the black hospital in Durham, and died minutes after his arrival. Durham's black newspaper concluded that he was another victim of "the carefully guarded segregation law of North Carolina that prohibited him being placed in any other space than that allotted for his race" (qtd. in Love 1996, 221). Duke University Hospital never publicly acknowledged that the segregation of its facility had caused the transfer. However, Duke's chairman of the Department of Medicine at that time, later reflecting about the hospital's policies, explained, "If there was no black bed available and if there were beds in the white service, he was sent somewhere else. Nobody sweated over it. It was just the era of segregated restaurants and toilets. It happened every day and some were bound to die" (qtd. in Love 1996, 224).

The Southern Conference Educational Fund published a report, *The Untouchables: The Meaning of Segregation in Hospitals*, in 1952. It described twelve cases, including Avery's, that led to death from being turned away from white hospitals whose black units were full or who refused all black admissions, including some in the North (Maund 1952). The cases took place over a twenty year period. Such events, or at least ones that would come to the attention of the media and be included in such a report, were rare for two reasons. First, at least in the South, the rules about where one could seek care or where ambulances would take you were clear. Only middle- and upper-class blacks with financial resources and a family member faced with a life threatening emergency were likely to challenge these exclusionary practices. For example, in 1946, 87.1 percent of white births and 45.2 percent of black births in the United State took place in hospitals. In Mississippi, the differences were event starker with 69.3 percent of the white births but only 9.6 percent of the black births taking place in such a setting (Dent 1949). In Mississippi the bulk of the out-of-hospital black births were attended by lay midwives at home. Few had any recourse to hospitals in the event of the need for a C-section or other emergency requiring hospital surgical facilities. The disparities in maternal and infant mortality rates reflected these differences and were largely just taken for granted. Second, as acknowledged in the Southern Conference Report, the number of beds allocated for blacks and whites in relation to their numbers was roughly equivalent even though their quality was not.[5] Only when the census of black patients was well above average were hospitals with segregated accommodations placed in a bind in terms of admission decisions.

The recollection of two people who grew up in the South and pursued health careers capture most of the oppressive nuances of the southern Jim Crow world of hospitals and health care.

Dr. Brenda Armstrong, who grew up in Rocky Mount, North Carolina, is now on the medical school faculty at Duke. She recalled her experiences in the 1950s with her physician father, Dr. Wiley T. Armstrong.

Meharry and Howard docs went back to the communities from which they came. My dad and uncle were GPs. Sometimes they just got paid in staples. My first memory of medical practice was going with Dad to deliver a baby in someone's home. He took me to help him stay awake. My sister and I were born at home. The hospital would not accept black patients. We had a birthing room in my house. My brother was born in 1956 with CP [cerebral palsy] because he was too big and needed to have a C-section. Although my mother was the wife of a physician, she could not be admitted to the hospital, even though my father pleaded with them. It was too late and risky to transport her all the way to the "Colored Ward" at Duke. As a result he was born at home vaginally, had a stroke and CP because of it. He could have been the brightest and most accomplished of us all. (Smith 1999, 32; Duke University Medical School)

Ms. Mattie Gadson grew up at the same time in Greenville, South Carolina, in a medical world that represented neither the worst nor the best of what the Jim Crow health care offered blacks.

If you needed hospital care, you went to the basement of Greenville General Hospital. It was Greenville's only hospital at the time. There was a separate entrance for blacks. I remember when I was in the first grade riding in a Harlem cab, one of the ones run by blacks for blacks. You couldn't ride in the yellow cabs; they were for whites. We were going up a hill it was slippery and we hit a utility pole. They took me to the emergency room at Greenville General. We were sent down to the basement to wait; it looked like a dungeon with pipes and everything. I waited and waited until all the white patients were seen. When I was older, I was hospitalized with a virus. They put me in an isolation room in the main hospital. I was really lucky. My aunt took in washing for the doctor who took care of me, so he arranged to put me in an isolation room on an all-white floor. I felt extra special, but my parents could only come at night to see me. I think it was because they did not want them to be seen on a white patient's floor. . . . Our family physician was Dr. Bailey; he had a black waiting room and a white waiting room. When he was finished with the white patients he would see you but as long as white patients kept coming in you got pushed further back. We did have a black dentist, however. I remember my first experience with a white dentist was when I went away to college. It was different. He had a separate entrance and waiting room for blacks. When I finally got to see him, he just pulled out pliers and yanked on the tooth. He didn't look to check to see if I had a cavity that needed to be filled or provide any pain killer, he just yanked it out. . . . My mom got cancer and by the time our doctor diagnosed it, it was inoperable. I remember I would go with her to the hospital clinic and the local mortician would provide the transportation with the understanding that when she died, he would get her body to prepare for burial. I didn't go to school on Wednesdays because that was her clinic day and I would go with her. The clinic was a cubby hole that they would pack the blacks; everyone in it was dying or half dead. They had a very nice waiting room for the whites. All the white patients in the white waiting room would be seen first. We use to go to the clinic at 9:00 in the morning and would not get out until 5:30 in the afternoon.

. . . In those days you really didn't realize you weren't getting the best of care. Any care was better than none. It was a just a way of life. I remember when my uncle's friend became Greenville's first black doctor in the 1950's. People in the black community flocked to his practice. He did home visits but I guess he didn't have any hospital privileges, because if you got admitted you had to be seen by a white physician.[6]

As a college student at Voorhees College, a historically black college in South Carolina, she participated in the voter registration drives in Mississippi in 1964.

I would see how terrified some blacks were to fill out the application. It was as if you were threatening their lives. They were afraid they would be kicked off the plantation and lose their livelihood. We did it anyway. This was a big thing then and everybody wanted to be a part of it. Everyone was concerned about human rights and today nobody gives a rip about human rights it seems. You had that inner feeling about being concerned about how people lived and how you could help them and their families have better lives.[7]

Ms. Gadson joined the tail end of the Great Migration that had begun fifty years earlier. She ended up in Philadelphia, serving for many years as a transplant coordinator at the Hospital of the University of Pennsylvania. That migration, beginning in 1915, brought almost six million blacks from the South to northern urban centers, where they struggled against different kinds of color lines.

The Great Migration and the Northern Color Line

"New things is comin' altogether diverse from what they has been" said this preacher in a rush of eloquence, and twenty voices of men and women shook out irresistible and magnetic melody to a song called "After a While." The last stanza ran like this:
> Our boasted land and nation is plunging in disgrace
> With pictures of starvation in almost every place
> While plenty of needed money remains in horrid piles,
> But God's going to rule this nation after a while,
> After a while
> After a while
> God's going to rule this nation after a while.
> (Sandburg 1919, 62)

Carl Sandburg's reports in the *Chicago Daily News* at the beginning of the summer of 1919 documented the rising tensions with the influx of southern blacks into the already overcrowded slums. Chicago was the epicenter of the Great Migration, and its black population had more than doubled during the First World War.

On the surface, never having a history of slavery and none of the trappings of Jim Crow, Chicago seemed, for those migrating from the Deep South, the Promised Land. State laws were passed after the Civil War that prohibited segregation of public accommodations and schools. Black people could vote and had for the first time the potential of acquiring real political power. Starting with World War I, the flow of low-wage immigrant workers from Europe was restricted. Chicago industries encouraged black migration from the South to address this shortage. For blacks from the Deep South, Chicago promised employment, better pay, and an escape from lynching and other acts of terror. Yet, as Walter Lippmann, influential liberal twentieth-century journalist and commentator, observed in the preface to a book of Sandburg's newspaper reports after the Chicago Riots of 1919, "Since permanent degradation is unthinkable, and amalgamation undesirable both for blacks and whites, the ideal would seem to lie in what might be called race parallelism. Parallel lines may be equally long and equally straight; they do not join except in infinity, which is further away than anyone need worry about just now" (Sandburg 1919, iv). Lippmann, just like most northern whites, embraced essentially the same "separate but equal" vision of white southerners, endorsed by the Supreme Court's *Plessy* decision. This involved the creation of a black ghetto to contain the migrants that would grow over the next fifty years to almost a million. Its boundaries were shaped by laws, public policies, and the profit motives of realtors and real estate investors. In the process, Chicago, as well as many other northern cities, became as racially segregated as any communities in the Jim Crow South. It could have worked out differently, but it didn't. The avarice of white realtors and the corruption of political leaders sustained the lie of separate but equal. It created a world for many of the migrants as brutal as any they had left (Simpson 2001).

In Chicago, tensions grew as the black migrants pressed against other working-class immigrant enclaves. In July 1919, a black teen had floated on a raft at the bathing beach across the imaginary line that marked the divide between the white and black parts of the beach. He was stoned by white boys, fell off his raft, and drowned. The police refused to arrest any of the perpetrators, and rocks began to be thrown from both sides. Violence spread, and by the end of three days twenty blacks and fourteen white men had been killed, and many homes of blacks were burned.

Racially restrictive covenants (also usually excluding Asians and Jews) subsequently controlled the spread of the black ghetto. In the 1930s these restrictive covenants placed almost 80 percent of the city's area off limits for black housing. The real estate practice of "block busting"—shifting all-white blocks to all-black ones, benefited the realtors and real estate speculators but no one else (Hirsch 1983, 1–38). The real estate interests profited from the white flight, buying up housing cheaply and then renting or selling it to blacks at inflated prices. Only in 1948, in the housing equivalent to the *Brown* decision on schools, did the Supreme Court rule that restrictive covenants were unconstitutional (*Shelley v. Kraemer*, 334 US 1 [1948]). That decision on housing was greeted with the same massive resistance that later greeted the *Brown* decision on public schools. In Chicago, homeowner associations, no longer able to legally enforce restrictive covenants, tried to pressure their members from selling or renting to blacks. When such pressures failed, violent intimidation by white neighbors tried to force black renters and homeowners out. These incidents were generally kept quiet by city officials and the media. They rarely involved forceful intervention by white police officers—unsympathetic to the new black residents—sent to keep the peace in these formerly all-white neighborhoods. Five residential areas of the city were the major battlegrounds, and a total of 319 arrests were eventually made of local residents for breaking windows, throwing fire bombs, and an assaulting the unwelcome newcomers (Hirsch 1983). Lorraine Hansberry's prize-winning play *A Raisin in the Sun* was based on her family's experiences. Her family battled the Woodlawn Property Owner's Association in a 1937 legal case that eventually led to the *Shelley* decision ruling that restrictive covenants were unconstitutional.

> The fight required our family to occupy disputed property in a hellishly hostile "white neighborhood" in which literally howling mobs surrounded our house. . . . My memories of this "correct" way of fighting white supremacy in America include being spat at, cursed and pummeled in the daily trek to and from school. And I also remember my desperate courageous mother, patrolling our household all night with a loaded German Luger [pistol], doggedly guarding her four children, while my father fought the respectable part of the battle in the Washington Court. (Hansberry 1970, 51)

While after World War II, arsons, bombings, and angry mobs typically greeted blacks seeking better private or public housing outside the overcrowded South Side ghetto, these incidents received little attention in the press or by politicians. An event in 1951, however, finally forced city and national acknowledgment of the problem. A black World War II veteran and graduate of Fisk University attempted to move into a rented apartment in the industrial suburb of Cicero. Local police tried to block him from moving his furniture in. They told him to "Get out of Cicero and don't come back in town or you'll get a bullet through you."[8] That evening the apartment building was surrounded by a mob of four thousand whites. They threw stones at the windows and set the building on fire. Twenty-one families housed there fled. Firemen that rushed to the building to deal with the blaze were pelted with bricks. Only when Governor Adlai Stevenson sent in National Guard troops, armed with bayonets, rifle butts, and tear gas, who cordoned off a three-hundred-yard perimeter, was some semblance of order restored. What really made this incident different from those that had preceded it, however, was that for the first time it was shown on television. The images produced national and international condemnation. Such coverage would play an increasing role in shaping the local and national debate over civil rights.

In spite of the violence faced by those seeking a place to live, the black population of Chicago continued to grow. By 1960, 816,000 blacks lived in Chicago. A *Look* magazine article in 1958 described Chicago as the most segregated large city in the nation, observing that "Chicago has no solution for segregation caused by prejudice and fear and the greed of some real estate operators and mortgagors" (qtd. in *Atlanta Daily World* 1958, 1). Chicago, as its black daily noted in despair, "has become a model bastion of resistance to integration. So long as the White Citizens' Councils and other segregationist aggregations can point to this city in the North as a shining example of successful segregation, so long will the South find inspiration in holding the line against racial equality" (*Chicago Daily Defender* 1960, 12).

Hospital and medical services in Chicago, not surprisingly, operated within the same color lines as the rest of Chicago. Residential segregation, financial incentives, medical staff privileging, and predilections of admitting clerks all combined to produce the same results. It was all invisible. There were no "smoking guns," and everyone could protest their innocence. As Quentin Young, MD, one of the leaders in the efforts to end discriminatory hospital practices in the city in the 1950s explained: "Doctors get their hospital staff appointments every year or two, at most every three years. While there is something that approaches tenure if you've been on a hospital staff for, say, twenty nine years without a blemish, doctors are not always courageous and they sure knew, with the ghetto encroaching, that it would be sacrilege to admit a black."[9]

The first efforts to pierce this half-century veil of innocence was a student-faculty campaign to end the exclusion of black patients from the University of Chicago Hospital and black students from its medical school in 1947. Returning veterans, members of the American Veterans Committee, an integrated veteran's association committed to racial desegregation and less pliable than typical undergraduates, responded to a complaint brought to them by a faculty member. He had tried to get a black domestic servant treated at the university's medical school hospital but was turned away. Jack Geiger, MD, one of the student activists, described the extreme pressure necessary to get the university to even acknowledge the problem.

> We ran some tests to confirm this practice, met with university officials (who stonewalled, beyond admitting that the Lying-In Hospital, on the record, refused to admit any blacks because it might upset the white patients) and then started interviewing and digging. We were aided by the fact that this was 1947, half the students were veterans, and half the secretaries in the university were veterans' wives (gender equality was not yet an issue) and we robbed their files at will. What that produced was 60 pages of documentation from their own files with some striking revelations: Lying-In; written instructions to admitting clerks at Billings on how to identify "black" addresses and callers and turn such people away; minutes of a medical school admissions committee in which members had recorded, about a black applicant, that "he's qualified but we're not ready to accept blacks yet," etc. We released the whole packet at a big student rally and press conference. . . . But still nothing happened.
>
> In early 1948, I tried a new tactic. I called Montague Cobb and went to see him at Howard, and we worked out a plan under which the best ten applicants to Howard Medical School would also apply to the University of Chicago. We explained to the UC Medical School that we would have copies of their transcripts, MCAT scores, references, etc., and that we would also get records of white veterans at UC applying to the medical school that year and matched pairs, grade point for grade point and MCAT for MCAT. . . .
>
> That made them nervous, but it was not what (finally) turned the tide—something I should have thought of much earlier. From the secretary of the university's vice-president for development (the

fund-raiser) we got a copy of his schedule; his next scheduled visit was to be in Pittsburgh, at Carnegie Mellon, to visit the foundation and to ask for some funds for some big capital project or other. We went there (again, an interracial committee of veterans from the student body) two days earlier, met with the foundation, handed them the 60 pages of documentation and said, in effect, that we weren't demanding anything but we thought they might want to consider whether they should give funds to a university that behaved like this. Four days later we got a call from the University Vice President, wanting to know what the group wanted the university to do. As I remember, the racial exclusions at the hospitals quietly ended and some blacks were finally admitted to the medical school that year. (Geiger 1999)

While this affected only the University of Chicago hospital and its medical school, it was the opening salvo of a twenty-year battle over the desegregation of Chicago's hospital system. In December 1949, a pedestrian hit by an automobile was taken to the Woodlawn Hospital, a private hospital located adjacent to the University of Chicago's campus. The hospital catered to its all-white medical staff and their private white patients. It would, on rare occasions, accept black emergency admissions but only if it did not require integrating a room with white patients. The victim, Trinidadian writer Eric Hercules, was held untreated in the emergency room for an hour and forty-five minutes and then transferred ten miles away to Cook County Hospital. Generally Woodlawn accepted blacks only as outpatients, and there were no beds available that would permit segregating Mr. Hercules in a room separate from the white patients. As the administrator explained, "I don't think we had a bedroom at the time. We could have set up a bed in the hall-way, but we did not want to assume responsibility for the man" (Maund 1952, 14–15). (Woodlawn could in theory have transferred him to the University of Chicago Medical Center next door, but evidently its professed changes in admission practices had not been communicated to them.) Mr. Hercules died of a fractured skull three hours later, a victim of the same fate that would befall Maltheus Avery a year later at Duke University Medical Center in Durham, North Carolina (Maund 1952).

The black patients of black doctors were restricted to the hospitals where they had admitting privileges. In Chicago this essentially meant either Provident, its historically black hospital, or Cook County, its public facility. Neither was a match for the expanding and more affluent private voluntary hospitals in Chicago that benefited from the growing private insurance coverage of their patients. These two hospitals faced serious financial constraints. Provident, a four-story two-hundred-bed facility, had but two toilets available on each floor.[10] Cook County operated on the nineteenth-century open ward model of charity hospitals, where there was little privacy and the more ambulatory patients helped in caring for the sicker patients to make up for the staffing shortages (Ansell 2011, 96–97).

The Committee to End Discrimination in Chicago's Medical Institutions formed in 1951 as an outgrowth of the earlier efforts to hold the University of Chicago Medical Center accountable.[11] The hospitals denied that they were involved in any discrimination, and some could even provide examples of blacks actually receiving care at their facilities. All the anecdotal evidence could easily be dismissed, and the committee needed a way to document the discrimination that was occurring more systematically. They asked the city commissioner of health for the birth and death records by hospital by race. The commissioner, Herman Bunderson, MD, an incorruptible curmudgeon who had faced down the Democratic machine and survived a long tenure as health commissioner, supplied them what they wanted. The numbers were remarkable. Of the fifty or so hospitals in the city, Cook County accounted for 80 percent of the black births and 50 percent of the deaths. Except for a handful of facilities, the other voluntary hospitals accounted for only a few black births and deaths. Quentin Young, MD, and his colleagues on the committee joked that "the only way that blacks showed up in the statistics for many of the city's voluntary hospitals were from births smuggled in in the wombs of white mothers and from deaths of emergency room patients who were ungrateful enough to die before they could be transferred."[12]

The hospitals acknowledged that the numbers were really bad but insisted that it was beyond their control. The numbers did, however, help convince the city council to pass ordinances making it illegal for hospitals to discriminate on the basis of race in their admissions and in the selection of medical staff. Nothing, however, changed, and for all intents and purposes, hospitals in Chicago remained just as segregated as those in the Jim Crow South. The barriers to such change remained as impenetrable in Chicago as they were in the South.

Indeed, it would have required unusual vision and courage for health care providers to do more than simply adapt to this poisoned environment. Even on the on the eve of Truman's executive orders desegregating the military and federal agencies, the VA hospital in Chicago was as segregated as the one in Jackson, Mississippi. At the Hines VA on the outskirts of Chicago blacks were restricted to one or two rooms on each specialty floor, and black veterans were turned away because there were "no more Negro beds." The practice had existed since 1918, when army surgeon general William C. Gogas, a native of Mobile, Alabama, ordered the segregation of its hospital wards and cafeteria seating arrangements of convalescent soldiers at mobilization camps in Texas. The federal government had supported the segregation and separate and unequal treatment of its military veterans in its own hospitals for fifty years. Why should private institutions set up to take care of their own do it differently than the federal government did in taking care of its own (*Chicago Daily Defender* 1918; *Atlanta Daily World* 1947)?

The Maturation of the US Health System

During the 1950s the US health system, a product of an era that enforced color lines in both the South and the North, reached maturity. Race, its most extreme physical and social division, was just one of many.

The indigent, regardless of race or ethnicity, were relegated to a separate system that included clinics with block scheduling and wooden benches and either the open charity wards of voluntary hospitals or the even starker accommodations in public hospitals. The voluntary hospitals, just as the public ones in the nineteenth century served only those without the resources for private care at home. By 1929, with the beginning of the first hospital health insurance plans (the voluntary Blue Cross plans developed by local community hospitals), the voluntary hospitals had begun to be transformed into doctors' workshops, essential to the practice of most specialists. At the same time, private voluntary hospitals became increasingly financially dependent on attracting doctors to their medical staff with paying patients. The arms war for the most up-to-date operating rooms, diagnostic equipment, and patient amenities designed to increase admission of paying patients was just beginning. New private rooms and floors for paying patients soon expanded into the bulk of accommodations in hospitals that originally functioned as charities. Hospitals went to great lengths to overcome the stigma of being just places for the indigent. The Hill-Rom furniture company, founded in the same year as the first Blue Cross hospital insurance plans, grew rapidly, providing attractive homelike hospital beds and furniture for the new private accommodations. Its annual revenue now exceeds two billion dollars (Hill-Rom 2014). By the 1950s, not only were most of the beds in voluntary hospitals on their private pay floors, but most of the larger ones had at least three different sets of china, silverware, and menus, visibly reflecting the nation's social class structure all under the same roof.

Hospitals also reflected all the racial and ethnic divisions of American society. Many hospitals were created to provide a place to practice or receive care for those discriminated against by the medical staffs of other hospitals. There were not just black and white hospitals but Protestant, Catholic, and Jewish ones, as well as Irish Catholic, Italian Catholic, German Jewish, and Russian Jewish hospitals.

The resulting fragmentation added to the cost, adversely affected the quality of care, and, eventually, undermined the moral authority of the medical professionals and private institutions whose power and control over the American health care system remained unquestioned throughout the 1950s. While professing to embrace the moral high ground—the duty to care for those in need and to prevent the exploitation of the vulnerable, white-majority hospitals and organized medicine consolidated their own power and succeeded in doing just the opposite. The health system that matured in the 1950s had three racially shaped features.

VOLUNTARISM

Government was excluded from any central role in its organization, financing, and regulation. A separate sector, a "voluntary" one operated neither by the government nor by the business sector, dominated all these functions.

Unlike other developed countries, the bulk of hospitals in the United States are voluntary, nonprofit ones. Most had their roots in charities set up to care for the "deserving poor" (that is, to take care of their own racial or ethnic group or at least ones that were seen as morally worthy of receiving assistance). The "nondeserving poor," which typically included most blacks, were relegated to the county and city facilities that had their origins in the poor farms and workhouses established originally as a form of punishment. Indeed, many such public facilities in the South served to punish emancipated blacks unwilling to continue working as sharecroppers on plantations and had continued to be distrusted by the black communities they served because of this.

The financing of health care was similarly dominated by voluntary organizations, controlled by these same white hospitals and professional associations. The nonprofit Blue Cross and Blue Shield producer cooperative insurance programs, established by local hospitals and medical societies, dominated the private health insurance market. Blacks were largely excluded from this market. The plans were based on employer group enrollment, and blacks were much less likely to be employed by an organization that provided such benefits. Even if they had such benefits, as the Pullman porters discovered in Chicago in the 1950s, they were less likely to be able to use them. Often the only option was to admit the porters and their families to Cook County Hospital. Chicago's public hospital for the indigent was a "nonparticipating hospital" for which the plan provided only five dollars a day.[13] Thus, not only were black Blue Cross subscribers limited in where they could receive hospital care, but they helped subsidize the more expensive care received by white subscribers at the voluntary hospitals that excluded black admissions.

Regulation of the quality of care in hospitals was also delegated to voluntary professional organizations. The Joint Commission on Accreditation of Hospitals, established in 1951, set the hospital standards. It was the outgrowth the voluntary self-improvement effort pioneered by the American College of Surgeons (ACS). The ACS hospital standardization program began in 1920 in an effort to forestall any government interference. "It is wise," the ACS argued, "that we lead now in a program for better care of patients rather than be forced later by the public" (American College of Surgeons 1920, 644). (Loyal Davis, one of the leaders of this effort, was Ronald Reagan's father-in-law and allegedly the source of many of his views against government regulation.) The Joint Commission on Accreditation of Hospitals represented all the white mainstream hospital and medical professional organizations.

The key component of the voluntary hospital standardization program was that every hospital had to have an organized medical staff that would restrict the use of the hospital to those who were admitted to its membership. This private voluntary body had absolute control over who used the hospital and how. Since hospitals still had charitable immunity from malpractice claims they had no need to interfere in the medical staff's business, at least as far as private paying patients were concerned. Many surgeons even used their own employees to assist them when doing surgery in the hospital. It was their workshop provided to them free of charge, and they could conduct their business in any way that its members agreed on. It was a private fraternal organization and one, of course, not immune from racial and ethnic prejudice nor economic self-interest in the selection of its members or the governance of them.

By 1950 white physicians and their medical associations had achieved total professional dominance over the American health system (Friedson 1970). They had a degree of autonomy in governing it unmatched in any other nation, where physicians had become constrained by service or employment contracts to national health insurance programs. It was not surprising that their medical associations attacked any encroachment of government that threatened their uniquely privileged position. Just as previous efforts, the Truman health insurance proposal had been attacked and defeated in a well-funded campaign that portrayed it as a step toward the tyranny of a totalitarian socialist state. The "voluntary" way was the American way (Poen 1979, 145). Indeed during the Truman administration enrollment in voluntary Blue Cross–Blue Shield programs had grown from twenty-eight million to sixty-eight million. The elderly, poor, and minorities, of course, were largely excluded. Proposals for the creation of the Medicare program would soon receive similar treatment. It was hard for black physicians and their patients to see much benefit from the absolute extra-governmental control of this "voluntary" system. Klan chapters and lynch mobs, after all, also exercised such voluntary extra-governmental control over them. If you don't trust the government to do what is right, why would you trust a voluntary organization that excluded you as a member or discriminated against you in providing services?

DUTY TO NEGLECT

The argument made for delegating control of the health system to private voluntary organizations and professional groups hinged not just on their unique expertise but on their adherence to a code of professional ethics that placed what was in the best interest of their patients and society as a whole ahead of their own interests. For hospitals and physicians involved in providing health care, the fundamental ethical principle was the "duty to care"—that those who needed care should get it. Certainly many physicians and hospitals provided free care to those who needed it but couldn't afford to pay (perhaps more so than now). No one defending the status quo in the 1950s in the United States or at any other time has ever been willing to concede that individuals really needing care didn't get it.

Yet, in terms of hard evidence, not only was that not happening in the 1950s; it had never happened in the history of modern medical care in the United States. A hard and fast iron rule had always governed the relationship between use of care and the need for it. Those that needed the most care, the poor and the disadvantaged ethnic minorities, got the least, and those that got the most, the more affluent and white populations, needed it the least. The differences in need for medical care were reflected in the mortality statistics that had been collected for half a century. In 1960 infant mortality rates (deaths per one thousand live births before one year of age) for black infants were 44.3, about twice as high as the 22.9 deaths per one thousand for white infants ("Infant Mortality Rates" n.d.). Age adjusted death rates per one hundred thousand blacks was 1,577.5, and for whites 1,311, making the black mortality rate about 20 percent higher (Centers for Disease Control 2014). Such persistent differences had been used by life insurance companies to charge higher rates to blacks or to exclude them altogether and, indirectly, by health insurers in targeting employer groups and geographic areas. The "smoking gun," the actual relationship between differences in mortality rates and differences in access to medical services, didn't begin to be reported on a national level until the 1960s. A pathbreaking effort to document differences in access to care by income during the early 1930s had excluded blacks because the study group concluded that they "could not procure satisfactory information from Negro families" (Falk, Klem, and Sinai 1933, 5). The statistics that began to be produced by the National Health Interview Survey in the 1960s documented stark differences in access by race and income. For example, in 1964, despite higher rates of morbidity and mortality, blacks had only 77 percent of the age adjusted physician contacts per year of whites, and low income persons had only 75 percent of the contacts of high income persons (Smith 1999, 202). Similarly age adjusted in 1964, blacks were only 75 percent as likely to be admitted to a hospital as whites, and low income persons were only 93 percent as likely as high income persons (Smith 1999, 203). Differences in access to preventive services such as regular physicals and immunizations were even greater, and, as has been suggested previously, crude counts understate the magnitude of the differences since the quality of these services differed as well. Care was provided inversely related to need whether by race or income and directly related to the ability of patients to pay for their care. That iron law had persisted throughout the half century of the development of the nation's modern medical care system. It was just the way things were, and few could envision it ever changing.

EXPLOITATION OF THE VULNERABLE

Blacks and the poor that lacked access to care were perceived by the white mainstream not so much as a problem in need of correction but as a useful resource for research and teaching purposes. Medical training and research at medical schools and teaching hospitals in the United States relied on this resource. If you did not have the ability to pay for care, you could exchange your body and ailments for research and teaching purposes for care. What was learned could then benefit the predominantly white paying patients and help train the physicians who would care for them. Most, both doctors and patients, involved in such exchanges felt uncomfortable about them—they were inherently exploitative.

Montague Cobb, Howard physician and physical anthropologist, who would later serve as the leader of the national hospital desegregation movement, observed that the Great Migration also included black cadavers that found their way on freight trains north in barrels labeled "Turpentine" bound for northern medical schools. With caustic irony he noted that the equality of the races, for the purposes of research and teaching, existed only after death (Cobb 1951).

The major public hospitals in the nation, such as Cook County, up through the 1950s were critical resources for medical schools and highly competitive sites for postgraduate medical training. In this context, the Tuskegee syphilis study was not something that would raise any ethical red flags. The rural Alabama blacks recruited for this study actually got care they would never have received even though no treatment was provided for their syphilis. Only after access to care greatly improved after the implementation of Medicare and Medicaid in the late 1960s did the study become a source of outrage and shame (Jones 1981). Before this, it was just taken for granted by the US Public Health

Service, by the national foundations that helped fund it, and by black as well as white medical professionals who lent their assistance. Paul Cornely, MD, Howard physician who became a central figure in the effort to desegregate hospitals, reflected in disbelief, "I spoke out for the racial integration of hospitals but I'm now not sure how forcefully I did this. It was a different time. I knew about the Tuskegee Syphilis Study. I ask myself now, why in the hell I didn't raise questions? I read about it in *Public Health Reports* in the late 1930s. I said, 'Mm this is really interesting.' Why I didn't raise that ethical point baffles me now but no one else did then either. I guess we all lost sight of those issues in the context of the times."[14]

That "teaching material" flowed with the Great Migration to northern cities such as Chicago. Quentin Young, MD, who trained at Cook County from 1947 to 1952 and later returned as chief of medicine, reflected on the nature of the institution.

> County as other public hospitals such as Kings County and Los Angles were still a central part of the model of physician training and one of the premier training centers. "Cook County hospital in the 1940's was not predominantly black. We had wards, about 3,300 beds in all and no control. You just added beds when you needed them. There were about 120 patients on a ward and an intern would be responsible for 60 inpatients and for admitting another 20 per day. There was very little support. We mixed our own penicillin. You had to fill vials with penicillin. There was esprit and culture to that group; it was like a battle zone. Attending positions were sought after. . . . It was all very much seat of the pants and not a place for liberals. A hospitalized person at County was either being punished by illness for being bad, the conservative position, or was the victim of poverty, lousy housing, and oppression, the radical view. You weren't judged for your politics you were judged by your outcomes. The good guys in terms of politics were not necessarily the best doctors. But, we had lots of shouting arguments. That is, was the mom hospitalized as a result of shooting up with heroin violating God's law and being punished or was she a victim of capitalist oppression? Well, both. God's a capitalist!"[15]

Rebellion

The more accepted mainstream narrative of medicine and health care in the first half of the twentieth century, of course, ignores the racial side of the story. It emphasizes the advances of medicine, the sacrifice of physicians in training in providing care to the indigent and the free care they provided in practice. It extols the role of voluntary hospitals and the voluntary insurance mechanisms in assuring that people had access to the care that they needed. It emphasizes the role of voluntary community hospital efforts in solving the access problems and assuring a high standard of care rather than insulating a white elite from public accountability. It emphasizes the efforts of medical schools and teaching hospitals to care for those abandoned by the mainstream of the medical care system. Most importantly, the conventional narrative contrasted the achievements of the "voluntary way" with the threat of totalitarian government control of socialized medicine (Poen 1979). That narrative, supported by the American Medical Association's well-funded public relations effort, blocked the passage of Truman's National Health Insurance bill in 1950. The facts presented here about segregated unequal access to care just got buried. As far as health care's mainstream narrative was concerned, race was invisible.

In its defense, medicine and health care in the United States didn't choose this any more than a child chooses its parents. It grew to maturity shaped by all the ethical inconsistencies, paranoia, and violence of the nation's racist past. A small group of black physicians and dentists, a minority of a minority with more backbone than was safe for them, would now force the nation's medical care system to deal with this.

Black medical professionals had all been on the losing end. While white mainstream voluntary hospitals might accept black patients, typically in segregated accommodations, they were far less likely to accept black physicians to their postgraduate training programs or their medical staffs. Subsequent activists Hubert Eaton, MD, and Paul Cornely, MD, were graduates of the University of Michigan Medical School, one of the early historically white medical schools to admit blacks. Yet blacks were excluded from the residency and specialty training opportunities available at the medical school's own hospital. Cornely eventually received an internship at historically black Lincoln Hospital in Raleigh-Durham, North Carolina. Excluded from any opportunities to pursue a surgical residency, he returned to the University of Michigan to receive training in public health and later began an academic career at Howard University, focused on eliminating hospital discrimination and segregation. Eaton obtained a residency at another historically black hospital in North Carolina, the Kate B. Reynolds Memorial Hospital in Winston-Salem, before setting up a practice in Wilmington, North Carolina.

Just like the first black physician in Greenville, South Carolina, in the 1950s, mentioned by Ms. Gadson, Eaton's practice thrived in an insulated world, providing a comfortable living, but at a price. Just as with others that would follow, one final insult pushed him over the edge, and the rebellion began.

> Before the call that summer day in 1947, I lived quietly and uneventfully. I had a thriving medical practice, a family that gave me pride and comfort, a home with a private tennis court. I . . . believed at 31 I was set on a satisfying, predictable course for my life. . . . Then the lawyer called. . . . He represented a patient of mine and needed my testimony in a dispute over the injuries incurred. The bailiff beckoned me toward the judge's bench.
>
> "Put your left hand on the Bible, raise your right hand and say after me." . . . I reached toward the shelf that stretched across the front of the judge's bench and saw two Bibles. Each had a strip of dirty adhesive tape on them. One was labeled "COLORED," the other "WHITE." Segregated Bibles. . . . Back at my office I got out of my car a different Hubert Eaton. In the years that followed . . . I changed my life and, I believe, my town. (Eaton 1984, 3–4)

After his epiphany with the segregated Bibles in a Wilmington courtroom, Eaton began a protracted legal struggle to win staff privileges for himself and other black physicians at Wilmington's white hospitals. He joined a small but growing band across the nation that had the backbone to lead a rebellion against all the pathologies produced in the American health system's formative years.

2

Backbone

Most people don't have the backbone to be rebels. The risks are too great and the price too high. Only a small minority became civil rights activists during the height of the civil rights struggle. So it was with the American Revolution, the resistance in Nazi-occupied Europe, opposition in Stalinist Russia, and the anti-Apartheid struggle in South Africa. Most people just kept quiet. Some flee as they did during the Great Migration to northern cities such as Chicago. Black physicians and dentists joined them, making those that stayed even more precious to the southern black communities they served. Most, however, sit on the sidelines, keeping their mouths shut, trying not to bring attention to themselves, and just trying to survive. A few out of fear or for personal gain collaborate with an oppressive regime helping to silence dissent. It takes backbone, perhaps even a little craziness, to stand up to overwhelming power. No backbone, no revolution.

Black health professionals supplied most of that backbone for the civil rights rebellion in the United States, for three reasons. First, just being medical providers, they were endowed with the same respect, authority, and autonomy that propelled the professional dominance of medicine as a whole in the 1950s. Second, since they were almost completely excluded from the white medical mainstream, they faced less risk of retaliation. Black physicians couldn't be kicked out of medical societies or off hospital medical staffs they were denied membership in, nor could they be severed from contracts with health insurers in which neither they nor their patients participated. Finally, the black communities these physicians served understood the economic insulation their patronage provided. Their patients demanded, in return, that they serve as their advocates.

As independent advocates for their patients, they were the embodiment of the ideal of organized medicine and hard to dismiss as communist sympathizers by the growing Cold War paranoia that helped spawn McCarthyism. After World War II the AMA and its local chapters fought to preserve and expand their dominance by embracing this ideal of independent fee for service practice against the intrusion of "socialism." Civil rights and universal health insurance advocacy got branded with the same brush. Organized medicine's campaign against the Truman National Health Insurance Plan included the distribution of a million copies of a pamphlet entitled "Compulsory Health Insurance—Political Medicine—Is Bad Medicine for America!" The pamphlet included the heartrending copy of the nineteenth-century painting by Sir Samuel Luke Fildes of *The Doctor* on a house call, devotedly huddled by lamplight over a sick child that included the heading "Keep Politics Out of This Picture!" (Poen 1979, 145). Ironically, the only physicians that still fit into that picture were black ones denied access to modern hospitals increasingly relied on by mainstream medicine. The AMA argued that "politics" meant "socialized medicine." At the same time local medical societies fought against early managed alternatives to fee for service. Depending on whether the sponsor was a labor union or a corporation it was labeled either "socialized medicine" or "corporate medicine." In either case, local medical societies labeled physicians participating in such plans as engaging in the "unethical" practice of medicine and denied them on this basis membership in local medical societies and privileges at hospitals. The fee-for-service practice of medicine was essential, they argued, in assuring that nothing get between physicians and patients in their essential role as their uncompromised advocate.

The profound irony was that, in organized medicine's advocacy for independent fee-for-service practice, black health professionals were not only excluded from membership but also made more effective in bringing about fundamental changes in the organization of health care. Indeed, if the AMA had not been so successful in assuring black physician autonomy, the black doctors would have been easier to control. The threat of economic sanctions might well have blocked their participation, and there would not have been a civil rights movement in medicine at all. In addition, these independent practitioners, as embodiments of the free market ideal, could never be convincingly attacked as part of a socialist/communist conspiracy. As a result, the AMA's campaign against the Truman National Health Insurance legislation helped strengthen the leadership role of black health professionals in the emerging civil rights movement and, eventually, in the struggle to pass Medicare and Medicaid.

Those who benefited from the efforts of these black health activists included more than just blacks. Other racial, religious, and ethnic groups faced similar discrimination in their practices. Not just black hospitals were created to adapt to these exclusions but also Irish Catholic, Italian Catholic, Russian Jewish, and German Jewish ones. Their mission was to take care of their own and adapt to the religious and ethnic exclusionary patterns of other facilities. Black physicians' efforts to break down the discriminatory barriers broke them down for everyone. More importantly, since many of their patients were poor, they became advocates for the indigent regardless of race or ethnicity. This would lead them and their national association into becoming the key medical advocates for greater federal government involvement in financing care and, eventually, into becoming the major medical supporters of the Medicare and Medicaid legislation.

If Medicare was the gift of the civil rights movement, it was in an exchange for the critical gift a few unusual health professionals provided the civil rights movement: backbone. Black doctors served as plaintiffs in many of the key cases involving school and other forms of segregation. They helped organize many of the boycotts, sit-ins, and other demonstrations in local communities. These medical civil rights rebels fell roughly into two groups—the street fighters and the Brahmins. The street fighters would challenge the white establishment through direct action—organizing demonstrations and boycotts. The Brahmin rebels would meet with professional groups to pressure change from the inside and bring lawsuits when this proved impossible. It was a division of labor, reflecting their personalities and class backgrounds that proved useful—one of many iterations of the "good policeman–bad policeman" routine that helped transform health care. It reflected the division of labor in the civil rights movement as a whole between the older civil rights groups, for example, the Urban League and National Association for the Advancement of Colored People (NAACP), and the younger groups more committed to direct action, the Southern Christian Leadership Conference (SCLC), Student Non-violent Coordinating Committee (SNCC), and the Congress of Racial Equality (CORE). The lives of three street fighters and three Brahmin rebels capture the story of the civil rights struggle to transform health care within the context of larger struggle.

The Street Fighters

Each of the street fighters had a Horatio Alger story: from humble beginning to prominence as a medical provider in the broader civil rights movement. All were irrepressible bundles of energy. They participated in all aspects of the movement, got their hands dirty in direct action, and, as the movement wound down at the end of the 1960s, were fortunate to just still be alive.

THEODORE ROOSEVELT MASON HOWARD, MD

Theodore Roosevelt Mason Howard (T. R. M.) had all the energy, brilliance, and oratory skills of his namesake, but none of his privileged background.[1] He was born in Murray, Kentucky, the son of a tobacco twister and a cook for a white doctor. T. R. M.'s energy and ambition impressed the doctor and Seventh Day Adventist. He put him to work at a young age in his hospital and then assisted in his education, which eventually led to a medical degree from the College of Medical Evangelists (now Loma Linda University). In 1942 he was appointed the chief surgeon of the new Taborian Hospital in Mound Bayou, Mississippi. The new hospital, established by the Knights and Daughters of Tabor, was a source of pride for the all-black Mississippi delta town. Such fraternal orders and lodges had served as a safety net for members before the creation of a public safety net. The Knights and Daughters of Tabor was established by freed slaves, and the hospital had been constructed with contributions from Mississippi members of the order. The hospital had been the brainchild of Dorothy Ferebee, a Tufts medical school graduate and one of the first black female medical school graduates in the country. As a faculty member at Howard Medical School, she had worked with Alpha Kappa Alpha, a black sorority, to set up health programs in the Mississippi delta, setting the stage for all the civil rights struggles that would follow. Just as other hospital cooperative insurance plans would evolve into regional Blue Cross plans, the operating expenses of Taborian were to be paid by dues (premiums). Dues for an adult were $8.40 a year, and that entitled the member to ninety-one days of hospitalization at the Taborian Hospital, including surgery and a $200 life insurance benefit. Mound Bayou was the parallel line of black development that Walter Lippmann referred to in his preface to Carl Sandburg's book on the Chicago Race Riot.[2]

Theodore Roosevelt Mason Howard, MD, fit right in. In addition to serving as surgeon in chief of the new hospital, Howard soon acquired controlling interest in the Magnolia Life Insurance Company, acquired extensive land holdings for cotton farming, and helped form the Regional Council of Negro Leadership (RCNL) in 1951. Through all these activities he nurtured the assertive, direct action leadership of the emerging civil rights movement. Medgar Evers, hired by Howard as an agent for the Magnolia Life Insurance Company, participated in the RCNL and was encouraged by him to take over the leadership of the NAACP. Aaron Henry, a pharmacist and operator of a drugstore in nearby Clarksdale, filled many of the prescriptions from Howard's Mound Bayou clinic, became a founding member of the RCNL and a lifetime civil rights activist. Howard hosted the annual meetings of the RCNL in Mound Bayou. He became acknowledged through these events as "the Modern Moses of Civil Rights in Mississippi." In 1955 it drew a crowd of more than ten thousand under a circus tent with more than three tons of barbecued chicken. The event included blues and gospel music singer Mahalia Jackson and featured speakers such as Thurgood Marshall and black congressmen from Chicago and Detroit. Howard's own spellbinding oratory pushed young blacks to buck the Jim Crow system. It was the civil rights equivalent of an annual Woodstock. The conference organized a boycott of gas stations that provided no restrooms for blacks and, more quietly, a campaign to register black voters. Most of the local NAACP chapters in Mississippi were formed by attendees transformed by the event, including Fannie Lou Hammer, who would later become a leader in the Mississippi Freedom Democratic Party.

In 1954, a few weeks before the Supreme Court's *Brown* decision, Thurgood Marshall provided the gathering with a hopeful message. The court's decision soon afterward was greeted with celebration by all the participants that had attended the RCNL meeting. The celebration was short-lived. As would be repeated many times, white leadership's willingness for reasoned accommodation to an end to the separate but equal legal divide soon gave way to a steely, ruthless backlash. The rapid consolidation of white resistance transformed Mississippi for its black citizens and those sympathetic to their cause into a police state as close to that of Nazi Germany and Stalinist Russia as experienced in the United States since the Civil War.

The white backlash to the *Brown* decision began over the summer of 1954. Local White Citizens' Councils, initially set up to block the desegregation of schools, broadened their attack. Sympathizers with desegregation got threatening phone calls, lost their automobile insurance, were unable to get loans, and had their taxes audited. "We won't gin their cotton, we won't allow them credit and we'll move them out of rented houses," one planter promised, and a state legislator suggested that "a few killings might save a lot of bloodshed later" (qtd. in Beito and Beito 2009, 97). Those sharecroppers who were patients of Dr. Clinton Battle, active in the RCNL and NAACP, were denied loans to pay him for his services. A blacklist of registered black voters was circulated, and it was made known that anyone who wanted credit or to keep his job better be off that list. Black voter registration in Mississippi plummeted from twenty-two thousand in 1954 to about eight thousand in 1956.

Howard, however, devised a strategy that helped blunt the economic threat. He developed mechanisms for black businesses, including physicians, to get their needed supplies from out-of-state vendors and set up a fund at the Tri-State Bank, a black bank in Nashville that he had business connections with, to provide credit to those businesses cut off from credit. Howard got North Carolina Mutual (the nation's oldest black life insurance company), the Brotherhood of Sleeping Car Porters, the Knights and Daughters of Tabor, and the United Auto Workers to contribute funds to support the Tri-State loan program. The countermoves were sufficiently credible that most white suppliers and loan companies backed off. The supply and credit squeeze abated. Howard knew how to use the power of the purse, and it would become a key weapon in the struggles that would follow.

The white backlash, however, marshaled all the weapons at its disposal. The Mississippi Sovereignty Commission in the governor's office coordinated the counterattack.[3] Its job was to fight local and federal efforts to desegregate schools and public accommodations and to block the registration of black voters by any means possible. They conducted an aggressive public relations campaign and investigations to undermine and discredit their adversaries. While some have tried subsequently to dismiss the activities of the commission as those of a bungling bunch of Keystone Cops, there is nothing humorous or amateurish suggested in their records, which were finally made public after protracted legal proceedings. Indeed, many subsequent police and privately financed political efforts against dissident groups have continued to operate using the same playbook. The FBI's own COINTEL-PRO (Counter Intelligence Program), established in 1956 at the same time as the Sovereignty Commission, used the same tactics against civil rights groups on a national level. The FBI and the commission shared information, and some of the commission's investigators were former FBI agents. COINTELPRO was dismantled in 1971 only after files revealing its existence and scope of operations were stolen by anti–Vietnam War activists from their Media, Pennsylvania, office and released to the press. The files of the Sovereignty Commission, shut down in 1977, became publicly available in 1998. How far the commission strayed into illegal activities, however, will never be known. On February 8, 1965, the Sovereignty Commission director ordered the purging of files of any incriminating information related to obstructing civil rights demonstration or voter registration and instructed investigators in their reports not to include anything that could raise legal challenges. (These instructions were ordered purged as well but, being a disciplined bureaucrat, the director sent a copy to the governor's office, which survived.) Yet what was left in its files was incriminating enough. The Sovereignty Commission helped fabricate crimes to imprison suspected civil rights activists and arranged for the termination of employment of civil rights activists, troublemaking university professors, and even college presidents. In more high-profile events, it assisted the legal defense team of Byron De La Beckwith providing information on potential jurors for his trial for the murder of Medgar Evers and provided the license plate number of the car ridden by civil rights workers James Chaney, Andrew Goodman, and Michael Schwerner to the sheriff of Neshoba County, who was implicated in their murders. The commission had a budget of about $2 million in current dollars, but, since it worked in close cooperation with all state agencies and local white citizen's councils, this understates its influence.

A key strategy used by the commission (also used by the FBI's COINTELPRO) was to hire informants inside the civil rights movement to provide intelligence, foment dissent, and undermine trust. Influential black community leaders—ministers, school officials, and newspaper editors—were among those widely known at the time to be paid by the commission for their assistance. This fostered the conclusion of many that there was no way that the civil rights movement could possibly win, so why not get on the winning side early. Besides, they would be working for the government so it had to be something perfectly legal that any good citizen would do. Moreover, lots of people could use a little extra money. The commission had no trouble recruiting informants. The most troubling disclosure from the public release of the Sovereignty Commission files, however, was revelation of the activities and identity of "Agent X." He was in a leadership position in the civil rights movement during the voter registration drives and Freedom Summer national civil rights efforts in Mississippi in 1964. He supplied the license plate number of the automobile used by CORE staffers that was pulled over by Neshoba County police near Philadelphia, Mississippi, on June 21, 1964. Murdered by the Klan, their bodies were recovered from an earthen dam forty-four days later. The news of their disappearance reached the Oxford Ohio Freedom Summer training sessions from where Agent X was providing daily intelligence reports. The governor of Mississippi dismissed concerns, suggesting that it was all a publicity hoax and that "they were probably in Cuba." He knew better as he indicated in a later interview (P. Johnson 1970).

Informant X also understood the danger and requested police protection on his return to Mississippi on June 26. The resulting request by the Sovereignty Commission director was acted on and passed on to the state police. Informant X was escorted home by Mississippi state troopers. His unsuspecting traveling companions were impressed by the "service" they received. Only after the commission's files were finally made public was existence and the identity of Informant X revealed. It shocked everyone in the Mississippi movement who had worked with him. R. L. Bolden had served as vice president of the Mississippi NAACP and later as head of the Mississippi Freedom Democratic Party. Informant X provided detailed information and listed all the participants at private civil rights group strategy sessions, but Bolden was never identified as a participant. Nor did the Sovereignty Commission, which kept records on all civil rights activists and those suspected of civil rights sympathies, have any reports on Bolden. Bolden died in 2012. Although acknowledging that he had worked for a detective agency hired by the commission, he insisted until his death that he wasn't Informant X. The scars from that betrayal a half century ago have yet to heal. None of these events would have surprised Howard, who in 1955 was certain that a well-crafted, violent backlash was coming.

Howard hit the peak of his recognition as a civil rights spokesperson in 1955, just as the full force of the white backlash in Mississippi was beginning. In August he went to the National Medical Association's annual meeting in Los Angeles to accept the honor of becoming its president-elect. This signaled not only national professional recognition, which as an isolated rural practitioner lacking the family pedigree and prestigious educational credentials Howard had not yet received, but also the final step in the transformation of the NMA into a civil rights organization. Back home, however, events were unfolding that would force him onto an even larger national stage where he would face far larger risks.

Emmitt Till, a fourteen-year-old from Chicago, was visiting relatives in Leflore County on the eastern edge of the Mississippi delta. On a dare he had flirted with a white woman in a grocery store. He was kidnapped, tortured, and murdered for this offense. When his maimed body was recovered from the Tallahatchie River a national media storm erupted. An all-white jury failed to convict the indicted defendants. Howard's fortified home in Mound Bayou had provided protection for witnesses and northern reporters. Armed caravans had driven them to the courthouse. Howard had overnight become a sensation as a speaker about these events on the lecture circuit. He gave a fiery speech in Chicago shortly after the recovery of Till's body. His picture and comments appeared prominently in the national black press. His speeches, previously only to relatively small black professional audiences, now attracted thousands. The crowds broke into open weeping and screams in hearing his accounts of Till's death.

The murders of civil rights activists in Mississippi began. Lamar Smith, who had worked on black voter registration, and Reverend George Lee, an official in the RCNL, both were gunned down. Gus Courts, the sixty-five-year-old grocer that headed up the Belzoni NAACP chapter and who was a speaker at the last RCNL gathering, was shot in front of his store. Although seriously wounded he avoided the local white hospital, got emergency treatment from Dr. Clinton Battle, another activist in the RCNL and NAACP. He later had surgery at the Taborian Hospital in Mound Bayou. After a long stay, he recovered. The first opportunity Howard had to vent his rage demanding a "freedom march on Washington" was to a rapt overflow crowd at the Dexter Avenue Baptist Church in Montgomery, Alabama. Its new twenty-six-year-old pastor, Martin Luther King, gave the invocation and benediction. Rosa Parks, a seamstress and NAACP official, sat in the audience. She recalled it vividly many years later as the first mass protest meeting she had attended. A few days later she refused to give up her seat on a bus to a white man, and a new stage of the civil rights struggle had begun.

King must have taken a good deal away from the session with Howard both in terms of concrete strategies and rhetorical flourishes. Unknown to both at the time, King would soon replace Howard as the movement's spokesperson.

One way or another, Howard's days in Mississippi were numbered. He lived with a Thompson submachine gun at the foot of his bed. His home was an armed camp, and his automobile had visible rifles and a concealed compartment with illegal high-caliber revolvers. He met threats with a response that the delta was on the edge of a bloody civil war. The threats were taken so seriously by the state legislature that strict gun control laws were proposed. In the midst of these rising tensions T. R. M. Howard, MD, was described by a CBS news reporter as the man with the shortest life expectancy in the nation. *Ebony* had published a list of eight civil rights activists in Mississippi who were the most likely targets of assassination. T. R. M. Howard, MD, headed the list. Seven of his RCNL colleagues were also included on that list. Two, George Lee and, later, Medgar Evers, were murdered. Another, Gus Courts, had barely escaped a shotgun assassination and relocated to Chicago. When shots were fired into H. McCoy's living room they barely missed his child. Dr. Clinton Battle, facing both economic and death threats, moved out of Mississippi. Emmett Stringer and T. V. Johnson, facing both economic blackmail and death threats, disengaged from civil rights activism and stayed. By the end of 1955 Howard and his family had relocated to Chicago. He had left Mound Bayou with much ambivalence and lived the rest of his life offstage and well outside of the national civil rights spotlight. The backlash had succeeded in forcing a retreat. It would be a long, difficult campaign requiring the courage and sacrifice of many more.

SONNIE WELLINGTON HEREFORD III, MD

In 1956, the year after T. R. M. Howard escaped from Mississippi to Chicago with his life, Sonnie Hereford III returned to his native Huntsville, Alabama, to set up a family practice.[4] Hereford had just finished his internship at St. Catherine's Hospital in Hammond, Indiana, in a white and relatively affluent area on the outskirts of Chicago, so the two almost passed each other going in opposite directions. For Hereford, it had been a difficult decision to make. His new wife had grown up in the North and was not anxious to be subjected to the Jim Crow South and its growing violence. The income of his practice there would at best be less than half of what he could earn from a practice in the northern outposts of the Great Migration. He knew the grinding poverty and overwhelming health problems he would face in the black community around Huntsville. He also knew the humiliation he and his wife would face there. At that time there was only one black physician serving a black population of more than ten thousand. None of the other black interns at St. Catherine's and few of his Meharry Medical School classmates had chosen to go back to the South. Hereford, however, had something to prove and felt drawn back.

His family had been sharecroppers, and his great grandparents, who died when he was about eight, had been slaves. The all-black school he first attended was surrounded on three sides by the city dump. The stench in the warmer months of the year could be overpowering. He walked seven miles to the school, passed by yellow school buses transporting the white children to their school. If they drove by fast he got covered in dust. If they drove by slowly, he got hit with rotten food and cussed at by the kids on the bus. He persevered and eventually managed to get accepted to Meharry Medical School, Nashville, Tennessee. Hereford got one of the slots Alabama helped support for black residents, since blacks were excluded from its own medical school. He graduated second in his class.

His Huntsville practice included many house calls to dilapidated shacks without plumbing. Soon he was responsible for as many as forty office visits and ten hospital visits a day. His active case load grew to almost five thousand. He charged what he felt his patients could afford, and many could not afford anything. He would sometimes try to reduce his fees by treating the entire family together at a discounted price. Such a pattern of practice would later raise red flags once a state Medicaid program was established but, during this period, was just a way to assure that people got the care they needed at a price they could afford.

Hereford faced the same racial exclusion from membership in the county medical society and to hospital medical staff privileges as elsewhere in the South. However, a special arrangement, like that for the other black doctor in Huntsville, was worked out for Hereford. While Hereford wasn't accepted for membership in the white county and state medical society or given privileges at Huntsville Hospital, necessity was the mother of invention. Many of the forty-five or so white physicians in the county proved to be helpful colleagues, even though most had segregated waiting rooms and were staunch segregationists. Several discretely assured him, "You'll get into the medical society soon. All we need are a few well attended funerals" (qtd. in Hereford and Ellis 2011, 74). The "special arrangement" for Dr. Drake, the town's other black physician, allowed him to admit patients to the "colored" wing. He also could come to medical staff meetings, but not as a voting member, and not to any social hour or meals that usually preceded the meetings, and only after all the meal trays had been taken away. At the meeting where Dr. Drake was to propose a similar arrangement for Dr. Hereford, he got there just a little too early and one of the waitresses made the mistake of pouring him a cup of coffee. Four white doctors stomped out, and Dr. Drake was taken aside and recommended to make his proposal for Dr. Hereford at another meeting. The colored wing on the first floor was composed of one large room that served as emergency room, delivery room, and operating room. Ten or twelve overflow patients could be accommodated in beds in the hallway. The second floor consisted of fourteen double-occupancy rooms and a four-bed postpartum room. Huntsville hospital was a public facility, owned and operated by the city, and thus not in a strong legal position to exclude black patients altogether. Hereford's presence attending his patients on the colored ward was tolerated as long as he was always polite to the white physicians and staff, sought to refer patients to them, and, most of all, was "invisible." Once at a case review meeting, some of the physicians questioned a white doctor's removal of the uterus of a black woman when other alternatives in terms of medication and monitoring seemed preferable. The doctor got annoyed by the questioning and sputtered out, "I just want to tell y'all something. Y'all have practiced in the South. The woman was an ignorant nigger woman, and you know no nigger woman gonna take her medicine and keep her appointments like you tell her to" (qtd. in Hereford and Ellis 2011, 59). That stopped the discussion, and the meeting proceeded to other matters. Hereford left the meeting feeling devastated for the woman and for his own invisibility.

Huntsville thought of itself as a progressive, growing community with none of the "Negro problems" that had produced the bus boycott in Montgomery, Alabama, which began in December 1955, or the lunch counter sit-ins that began in Greensboro, North Carolina, in February 1960. That all changed in February 1962. Up to that point, Dr. Hereford's only civil rights act had been to register to vote in September

1956 just before opening his practice in Huntsville. Just as in other cities, however, anger over accumulating Jim Crow indignities were about to explode. The spark that ignited the firestorm of local community protest was Hank Thomas, CORE field agent who showed up first at A&M College and then at the black high school. Thomas recruited students to join him in a sit-in at downtown lunch counters. The students were arrested, fined, and jailed. A mass meeting followed at the First Baptist Church, led by Reverend Ezekiel Bell, and the Community Service Committee (CSC) was formed, with Hereford and a black dentist participating in its strategy sessions. (The other two black physicians practicing at the time in Huntsville steered clear of any involvement in the civil rights protests.)[5] All segments of the black community in Huntsville were involved. The campaign benefited from the lessons learned in earlier protests elsewhere. They kept the demonstration pressure on in the downtown movie theater and lunch counters, demanding the formation of a biracial committee to plan the desegregation of public accommodations. The marchers created signs that read "Are you shopping for freedom or buying segregation?"; "Khrushchev can eat here but I can't"; and "Rocket City: Let Freedom Begin Here."

The demonstrators, jailed for trespass, were stonewalled by the mayor, city council, and local paper. However, massive federal funding was flowing into Huntsville's Redstone Arsenal and to the NASA Marshall Space Flight Center. The Cold War race with the Soviets to develop nuclear intercontinental ballistic missiles and for space supremacy had transformed Huntsville into a boom town. The demonstrators wanted to get Huntsville in the national spotlight and thus threaten the flow of federal funds. A visit by Martin Luther King with an impromptu parade around Huntsville in Hereford's new Cadillac convertible was capped off with a mass meeting at Oakwood College, where King described how expensive the perpetuation of Jim Crow was going to be for Huntsville. The "expensiveness" that all sides in Huntsville were concerned about was potential loss of federal dollars flowing into the city's space and defense projects. The local newspaper, however, refused to cover the protests and tried to bury the story. National news outlets didn't cover stories not covered by local papers. That ended only after Hereford's wife, seven months' pregnant, and the wife of a black dentist, John Cashin Jr., with their four-month-old infant, joined one of the sit-ins and were jailed. National media covered the story, and the local paper was forced to cover it as well. Shortly afterward, a four-person interracial committee formed. The secret, staged plan they developed peacefully broke down all the color barriers in public accommodations within a year. By the time Johnson signed the Civil Rights Act in 1964, Huntsville was in full compliance.

In the midst of all the sit-in protests, never drawing any public attention, Huntsville Hospital was integrated. Hereford was assigned to a subcommittee of one of the CSCs to negotiate the desegregation of the hospital. He met with the administrator and was taken aback, expecting to be stonewalled. Mr. Larry Rigby, the administrator, said, "Dr. Hereford, I can see it coming. I know we're going to have to do something. Let me just think this over for a day or two and you come back, and we'll meet again, and I'll tell you what I've decided, and you can tell me whether you and your committee will be pleased with that" (qtd. in Hereford and Ellis 2011, 111). At the second meeting the administrator said, "I'll tell you what I've decided and you tell me what you think about it. In about two or three weeks I'll just quietly walk over one morning, and tell the nurses in the newborn nursery to accept black babies. And then, after that has soaked in, and they get used to that, we'll integrate labor and delivery and the post-partum ward. And assuming things go just fine, we'll do medicine. And then we'll do surgery" (qtd. in Hereford and Ellis 2011, 111). Hereford and the CSC were relieved that no protests would be required to pressure the hospital. Mr. Rigby did just as he said he would, walked over and told the nurses running the new born nursery, "We're gonna have all the babies born today and from now on, you accept them" (qtd. in Hereford and Ellis 2011, 111). In twelve months the hospital was completely integrated, including its cafeteria. The first few months in the integrated cafeteria were tense, but soon all the black and white nurses from the same units were sitting at the same tables, eating and laughing together.

The integration of most hospitals in the South didn't happen nearly as quickly nor as smoothly. Why was Huntsville Hospital one of the few exceptions? Certainly the intelligent leadership of the administrator in implementing the desegregation plan of the hospital played an important role. It was not, however, his decision to make. Why did the medical staff, still dominated by dyed-in-the-wool segregationists who regarded the hospital as their fiefdom, acquiesce? Why did the hospital's board, typically key powerbrokers in the city, meekly roll over? The hospital's white patients and their families just didn't have an instant magical conversion to racial justice. Why did they put up with it?

The exceptions, such as Huntsville Hospital, help to explain the persistence of segregation in most hospitals. First, the hospital was a public one, owned by the city of Huntsville. Its board was appointed by elected city officials. Public facilities faced legal pressure to integrate that private voluntary hospitals, at least for the time being, eluded. More importantly, those public officials had, as a result of the protests, chosen to integrate public accommodations in Huntsville rather than risk the loss of federal funding. The hospital board those public officials appointed would, understandably, acquiesce. Second, for the hospital's medical staff that already treated blacks and had gotten used to working with black physicians such as Dr. Hereford in the hospital, it was not a major adjustment. They would, of course, be concerned about the impact the change might have on their patients. That, as it turned out, was not much of a problem either. Huntsville Hospital was the *only* hospital in the area, and there could be no possibility of white flight. Patients and their families also gave much more deference to their physicians then and accepted their decisions. If their doctor admitted them and said it was OK, and, indeed if they had no other choice, it would be OK. Even though the hospital was integrated, it would try to accommodate their preferences, and some racial matching of rooms probably continued. Those practices would come to an end soon through federal intervention.

The final and most traumatic hurdle for Huntsville was the desegregation of its public schools. After a federal court order on September 3, 1963, Hereford marched, holding the hand of his five-year-old son, to the Fifth Avenue Elementary School. They were met by a mob and state troopers sent by Governor George Wallace. The troopers turned them away along with all the white students. Similar scenes greeted those attempting to integrate schools under the same court order in Mobile, Tuskegee, and Birmingham. Wallace had made his challenge clear earlier, on January 14, 1963, in his inaugural speech in the portico of the state capitol, where Jefferson Davis had been sworn in to the presidency of the Confederacy: "In the name of the greatest people that have ever trod this earth, I draw the line in the dust and toss the gauntlet before the feet of tyranny, and I say segregation now, segregation tomorrow, segregation forever" (Wallace 1963).

Martin Luther King would set the stage for Hereford, responding to Wallace's earlier challenge on August 28, 1963, at the Lincoln Memorial in Washington, DC: "I have a dream that one day, down in

Alabama, with its vicious racists, with its governor having his lips dipping with the words of 'interposition' and 'nullification'—one day right there in Alabama little black boys and black girls will be able to join hands with little white boys and white girls as sisters and brothers" (King 1963).

Wallace had helped unleash a wave of violence that included the bombing of the Sixteenth Avenue Baptist Church in Birmingham on September 16, 1963, which killed four young girls, a little over a week after Hereford had tried to enroll his son in school. He and his son were in the eye of the storm. Hereford had been getting constant threatening calls from the KKK at his office and home. He found the best way to answer them was to say, "This is the Hereford residence, Officer Parker speaking . . . if it was a threatening call, you'd hear a click" (Hereford and Ellis 2011, 116).

Yet, mysteriously, the storm abated. The following Monday Hereford with his son walked again to the school. The crowd had disappeared, and so had the state troopers. As *Newsweek* would later describe the event, "A wide-eyed first grader, Sonnie Hereford IV, his hand clasped in that of his father, Sonnie Hereford III, had walked unhindered into a Huntsville elementary school to become the first Negro to break the grade school color barrier in Alabama" (qtd. in Hereford and Ellis 2011, 118). Wallace's state troopers remained on duty to block entrance to the schools in Birmingham, Mobile, and Tuskegee. What had happened? One has to assume that the white leadership in Huntsville feared loss of federal funds for Redstone Arsenal, and desegregating the schools was a price they were willing to pay to keep that funding. That message had gotten to the governor, and he backed down. The power of the federal purse or just the threat of its use by civil rights activists had carried the day.

History never lacks in ironies. The Huntsville Redstone Arsenal at the height of the Cold War employed German defector Werner von Braun. His team at the arsenal developed the first rockets used for nuclear ballistic missiles. During World War II von Braun had worked on the German missile program. He became an SS member, and his missile program used slave labor from concentration camps. Hereford's son, who became the first black student to integrate an elementary school in Alabama, later worked as a software engineer at the same center in Huntsville. Thus, the same federal dollars that supported von

Braun's work forced Wallace's tactical retreat and Hereford's son's desegregation of the public school and provided his subsequent employment (Sonnie Wellington Hereford IV 2007).[6]

REGINALD HAWKINS, DDS

Reginald Hawkins, DDS, made a career out of being a far more persistent and confrontational street fighter than either T. R. M. Howard or Sonnie Hereford III. In part, he learned his militancy was necessary to accomplish change in the large and growing city of Charlotte, North Carolina. Charlotte was led by a white business elite and chamber of commerce concerned with luring new companies by promoting a business-friendly progressivism and an illusion of racial harmony.

In part it was just a matter of temperament. Born in Beauford, a small fishing village on the Inner Banks of the North Carolina coast, he came from a family that placed much importance on backbone. His father's family had been pioneers in setting up black churches and colleges and had produced activist pastors. His father was employed by the US Department of Interior and did fish culture and ecological surveys along the eastern seaboard. His mother, a Croatan Indian, taught him at an early age to defy segregation and never grow accustomed to it. He did so for the rest of his life.

Hawkins left Beauford in 1941, to attend Johnson C. Smith College in Charlotte. He was quarterback on its football team, became a collegiate champion wrestler, and boxed competitively on the side. His aggressive instincts were not limited to contact sports. He became president of the student council and was active in early civil rights efforts to force the Charlotte post office to hire blacks and to organize a student boycott of a discriminatory dry cleaners near campus, forcing its closure.

In 1944 he was admitted to dental school at Howard University and soon found himself in the midst of many of the architects of the looming civil rights revolution. He was included among those that met on Sundays for a seminar on constitutional rights directed by Charles Houston, Thurgood Marshall, Jim Nabrit, Spottswood Robinson, and Leon Ransom. "After the seminar we would go down and sit in at Peoples Drug Store or picket the National Theater and Constitution Hall where Marion Anderson was denied the right to sing."[7] He also came under the wing of Montague Cobb, MD, who became the architect of the hospital desegregation movement. They would continue their relationship for the rest of their careers. At Howard, he had become part of an activist inner circle.[8]

He returned to Charlotte to set up his practice in 1948, indoctrinated in a way few dentists have ever been. On his return to Charlotte he was welcomed into the fold of the local NAACP by its president, Kelly Alexander. There were, however, white dentists on the local draft board, and even though he had been deferred because of being declared essential as the only black dentist doing oral surgery, they, according to Hawkins, were instrumental in getting his classification changed so he was inducted. Before being shipped off, however, he helped organize a sit-in to protest segregation of blacks and American Indians at the city's airport, the first sit-in in North Carolina.

Hawkins never missed an opportunity to push his desegregation agenda and used his induction to good advantage. He was sent to nearby Fort Bragg and proceeded to work with those responsible for its desegregation after President Truman's executive order. The general in charge of the base delayed implementing any changes. Hawkins used a special tactic to break the general's intransigence, unique in the history of the civil rights movement:

> The general was quite racist coming and going. He did everything he could to intimidate me. I was responsible for getting troops combat ready to be shipped overseas. That meant assuring no one had any dental problems. So I went with all my brigade to do an inspection. I looked in his mouth and said, "General, I hate to say this, but all your teeth have to come out. I want you in my clinic Monday morning. That's a direct order." The General jumped and said, "I got the message!" That's how I integrated Fort Bragg.[9]

At Fort Bragg his roommate, a rabbi and psychiatrist, convinced him that there was no way he was going to be able to do anything in civil rights without religion. When he returned to Charlotte he added a divinity degree from John C. Smith Seminary to his weapons. It became an important part of his life, and he served as pastor intermittently.

The Brown decision helped propel local actions that supported Charlotte's image as a progressive southern city. The Mecklenburg County Medical Society became the first local society in North Carolina to desegregate professional membership in 1954, a decision that ultimately forced the integration of the state society. Public libraries and some other public accommodations were also desegregated at this time.

Hawkins, however, became increasingly convinced that direct action rather than interracial committees and legal proceedings in the courts were the only way to achieve real change. You had to embarrass the white business elite and chamber of commerce concerned with luring new businesses to Charlotte. Business didn't move to places, such as Birmingham, that were getting a reputation for racial conflict, so Hawkins believed you had to create some to force real change. Much of his efforts focused on desegregating the schools beyond just tokenism. Protests, in addition to a legal suit, pushed this agenda. In 1961, he organized a black boycott of a school at the same time that Charlotte was planning to host the North Carolina World Trade Fair. Hawkins announced that "all was not fair in Charlotte" and proceeded to ignore warnings from the white leaders against causing embarrassments during the fair. "What do they know about embarrassment," he said, "we've been embarrassed all of our lives" (qtd. in Douglas 1994, 722). Hawkins won the concessions he wanted from the school board and called off the school boycott and disruption of the fair. He favored confrontation with the more bigoted elements of the community instead of negotiations with the white elite, which he dismissed as "having to go with clean fingernails and begging" (qtd. in Richardson 2005, 356).

In terms of health care in Charlotte, Hawkins's assessment appeared to be correct. Despite protestations of good intentions, the hospitals still remained segregated in 1963. Charlotte Memorial, a public facility recently expanded and renovated with federal Hill-Burton funds, had 475 beds with only thirty-eight allocated to blacks. Of the city's two private voluntary hospitals, Mercy Hospital had allocated thirty-two beds for blacks, and Presbyterian Hospital excluded them altogether. That left Good Samaritan, the oldest historically black private hospital in the country, with an aging physical plant that had not been upgraded even though the city had assumed full ownership of it in 1961. Adding to the concern of the students at John C. Smith, one of its football players had died at Good Samaritan after surgery for an injury during practice in 1961. The more updated facilities and equipment at Memorial might have prevented his death. Memorial offered as a concession an additional twenty beds in a new wing being constructed. As far as Hawkins was concerned the war was still on, and appeasement by allocation of Negro beds wasn't the answer. The John C. Smith students began picketing all the hospitals in Charlotte under Hawkins's guidance in March 1962. Their picketing of downtown hotels, restaurants, and theaters also resumed. The typical signs they carried included "This Hospital is built on the Rock of Segregation"; and "Is this Christian tradition? Segregated hospitals?" (Cobb 1964b, 228). The mayor dismissed the picketing as "belligerent acts of pressure" and said the students had "resorted to coercion, instead of lending support and cooperation to the community leadership" (qtd. in Richardson 2005, 366). An editorial in the local paper dismissed the picketing as "hysteria" (qtd. in Richardson 2005, 366). In response, on Sunday, March 24, 1962, sixty students and others, including a half dozen whites, held a fifteen-minute prayer service on the front lawn of Memorial Hospital.

These actions, some of the only recorded public picketing to pressure hospital desegregation ever to take place in the United States, helped to make Hawkins persona non grata in any joint collaborations with the white business leadership of Charlotte. It also deeply divided black leadership between those favoring the more traditional approach by the NAACP of negotiation with white leaders and the pursuit of remedies in the courts when this failed and that of a newer brand of leaders favoring broader direct action. In addition, many of the black physicians were concerned with assuring a strategy for the survival of Good Samaritan, which was their clinical home. Desegregation of all of Charlotte's hospitals, they feared, would result in the demise of Good Samaritan, an institution with a proud history in Charlotte's black community.

None of this deterred Hawkins. When in June there was still no movement, Hawkins played his best card. A letter sent by Hawkins to Attorney General Robert Kennedy demanded an investigation of Memorial Hospital's compliance with the nondiscriminatory provisions of the Hill-Burton Act. Three public health services officers visited Memorial on August 15, 1962. That same day the hospital's administrator announced, with no specifics, "The doors are open to any and all." After another year and a second visit by the Public Health Service officials, the hospital's board announced a new open-door policy in which it declared, "It can be assumed that Memorial Hospital will begin immediately to apply the same admission policies to Negro as white patients." In March 1965 Presbyterian Hospital, a private hospital planning a major expansion and Charlotte's last remaining all-white hospital, announced plans to admit blacks (Conn 1965).[10]

Hawkins's tactics accelerated the hospital and medical integration process in Charlotte. Like other street fighters, however, he faced threats of violent retaliation for his actions. In spite of Charlotte's business leaders' efforts to portray the city as progressive, one ruled by racial civility, Hawkins came the closest to losing his life, as did his colleagues Julius Chambers, a civil rights lawyer bringing the school desegregation suits, and two leaders of the local NAACP chapter, Kelly Alexander and Fred Alexander. On November 22, 1965, "night riding terrorists" threw sticks of dynamite into Hawkins's home and the homes of three other Charlotte civil rights activists. No one was ever arrested. For Hawkins, it just came with the territory occupied by a street fighter:

> It was planned. It wasn't any simple minded Ku Klux Klan
> operation. We know who did it. The FBI was more against me
> than those that did the bombing. They bombed us within three
> minutes of each other—me, Julius Chambers, Fred Alexander and
> Kelly Alexander. All our homes were bombed. They knew exactly
> where we were. It was lucky none of us were killed. . . . I was shot at
> thirteen times, my office was smeared with red paint. They bombed
> Julius's car and set fire to his office on Tenth Street. . . . It was
> serious. They were trying to kill us. They first tried to intimidate me
> and buy me off. They would come in my office with suitcases full of
> money. I'd tell them, "Get out of here."[11]

The pressures toward desegregation, however, were converging. In his battle to desegregate Charlotte Memorial Hospital, Hawkins was now taking advantage of the backbone and quiet persistence of another group, those working on a larger national stage: the Brahmin Rebels. The two streams of civil rights protest were coming together.

The Brahmin Rebels

If there is anything more uncomfortable to talk about in the United States than race, it is class. Class divisions existed in the civil rights movement and medicine, just as everywhere else. The NAACP, the Urban League, and other older civil rights groups grew out of early civil rights efforts that emphasized civil discourse between black and white leadership and orderly pursuit of remedies in the courts when such discussions failed. Their memberships were middle-class professionals with leadership often from prominent families. The newer, post–World War II direct action groups, Congress of Racial Equality (CORE), Southern Christian Leadership Conference (SCLC), and the Student Non-violent Coordinating Committee (SNCC), were democratically participatory organizations offering membership for anyone who would show up on the picket lines or at lunch counter sit-ins and face beatings and jail time. No college degree was required. They were organized in local churches, colleges, high schools, and fledgling labor unions. College and high school students played central roles. For example, students at North Carolina A&T in Greensboro started the sit-in movement, and Alabama A&M and high school students started the protest movement in Huntsville.

These same class divisions were reflected among the medical activists. The approach of the "Brahmin" rebels, in contrast to the more youth-driven street fighters, reflected their class background. The Brahmins were restrained, courteous to a fault, and models of respectability that preferred low-keyed negotiations and orderly court proceedings. Yet only when the two streams of activism joined in the early 1960s, despite the discomfort of both groups, did they become an effective force.

W. MONTAGUE COBB, MD, PHD

W. Montague Cobb, MD, PhD, served as a pall bearer for Charles Drew, a Howard medical school colleague who was killed in a car crash in 1950. Segregation faced by black travelers in the South contributed to his death from an automobile accident in North Carolina. Cobb had been a close friend and classmate at Dunbar High School in Washington and at Amherst College, as well as a colleague at Howard's medical school. Those credentials along with his PhD in physical anthropology, highly regarded scholarship, and chairmanship of the Anatomy Department at Howard set him at the top of his profession and promised a comfortable, privileged life with time for his favorite hobby, playing the classical violin.

Cobb, however, had backbone more than matching any of the street fighters. There would be no passive acceptance of any aspect of second-class citizenship in exchange for comfort. As a Brahmin rebel he had two important weapons in his arsenal.

First, his pen was sharper than any sword. As a young professor of anatomy at Howard in 1947, he got off to a rocky start in black medical society politics. He wrote a commentary on the annual national meeting of the National Medical Association (NMA) in Los Angeles in the Washington black medical society's bulletin (black physicians had yet to be accepted in the local chapter of the American Medical Association): "If an organization exists because of the fact of racial exclusion and fails to compensate for the effect of that exclusion or fight the discrimination itself, what purpose does it serve?" Cobb asked. He dismissed the final business meeting of the House of Delegates "as a colossal waste of time, major issues like financial provisions for medical care and measures against discriminatory practices in medicine received only the barest attention by the remnant of a very fatigued group" (qtd. in Smith 1999, 48). This outburst was picked up by the Associated Negro Press and reproduced in many black newspapers across the country, much to the consternation of the NMA's officers. Cobb refused to back down and apologize. In an act of good judgment, rare in the leaders of professional associations who feel their competence is being questioned, they appointed Cobb editor of the *Journal of the National Medical Association* in 1948, getting him to point his sword at the real adversaries. This represented a significant shift in editorial policy from a more conservative separate development focus. Cobb replaced John A. Kenney Sr., MD, who had been editor for thirty years and, perhaps more tellingly, who was the personal physician of Booker T. Washington early in his career.[12] The first step taken by the new editor was to add a regular feature to the journal, "The Integration Battlefront." The campaign to desegregate health care was just beginning, and Cobb, by implication, was its commander.

The other weapon in Cobb's arsenal was a tightly knit network of young black medical professionals who shared his vision. A highly regarded teacher, he taught almost six thousand medical and dental students, most of them African American, during his career at Howard. Many of these former students would serve in key roles in Cobb's campaign to desegregate the nation's hospitals. He worked in collaboration with Reginald Hawkins, for example, who had come under his wing as a dental student at Howard.[13] It was Cobb who had directed his attention to a provision in the Hill-Burton Act that, through Cobb's pressure, had led to the visit to Charlotte Memorial by the Public Health Service team.

Cobb, in directing this campaign, quickly forged an alliance with the NAACP. In a 1953 speech to the annual meeting of the NAACP later reproduced in the *Journal of the National Medical Association*, he called his troops to battle:

> As a logical step in its program to make the benefits and responsibilities of full citizenship available to all Americans, the National Association for the Advancement of Colored People today embarks upon a campaign to eliminate hospital discrimination in the United States. This will be a long campaign, sure to be marked by reverses as well as victories. But let us remember William Tecumseh Sherman, one of America's greatest generals. He never won a battle, but never lost a campaign. . . . The strategic focus of attention must be upon hospital discrimination for it is from this that the greatest harm results and it is in this area that the NAACP, as a lay organization, can play its most effective role. . . . The notorious basement ward for colored patients must be eradicated. But along with it must go the separate wards of all types, the relegation of Negro patients to the oldest and outmoded buildings, . . . the disruption of the sacred doctor-patient relationship effected when a Negro physician must leave his patient at a hospital door because he cannot be a member of the staff. . . . The subtle economic exploitation of the Negro by white physicians and institutions through racial bars in hospitals must be brought to an end. (Cobb 1953, 333–37)

Cobb's campaign, much to the irritation of most of the southern white medical establishment, certainly was Sherman-like. May 17, 1954, the date of the *Brown v. Board of Education* Supreme Court decision, he announced, "takes its place in the annals of freedom alongside the dates of the Fourth of July, which commemorates the signing of the Declaration of Independence of the American Colonies in 1776 and the Fourteenth of July which commemorates the storming of the Bastille in 1789" (Cobb 1954, 269).

In truth, the campaign to desegregate hospitals divided the rank-and-file members of the NMA, and Cobb was off the leash that typically holds an editor of a professional journal to middle-of-the-road positions. Many, probably a majority, doubted that the desegregation campaign would be successful and wanted the NMA to focus on the more pressing need to support a financially stressed black hospital system. The skeptics knew from bitter experience how insulated the historically white hospitals were from such pressures. Most were private voluntary institutions, insulated in a way that local publicly owned hospitals such as Huntsville and Charlotte Memorial were not. Indeed, they had been created and designed to resist public pressure and intrusion by government regulators. They placed a high value on the professional autonomy of their medical staffs. Their boards, selected for their wealth and influence, helped assure that autonomy and operated behind closed doors.

However, those doors had opened a crack as a result of the *Brown v. Board of Education* decision. The 1946 Hill-Burton Act had provided most of the nation's hospitals with federal matching funds for construction and renovation. These funds were allocated on the basis of need as determined by a state plan. However, the act's coauthor, Lister Hill (D, AL), who would later sign the southern manifesto pledging massive resistance to the *Brown* decision, inserted in section 662(f) of the act a statement that the recipient of funding must assure that "such a hospital or addition will be made available to all persons residing in the territorial area of the applicant without discrimination on account of race, creed or color *but an exception will be made in cases where separate hospital facilities are provided for separate population groups if the plan makes equitable provision on the basis of need for facilities and services of like quality for each such group*" (italics added). This "assurance" was the only explicit acknowledgement that federal funds could be used in a way that discriminated on the basis of race appearing in any twentieth-century federal legislation. Cobb's group launched a three-pronged attack focused on the Hill-Burton separate but equal provision seeking: (1) voluntary hospital desegregation through an appeal to reason and fairness, (2) legislation that would revoke the Hill-Burton exemption, and (3) a federal court ruling that would declare the exemption unconstitutional.

The first prong involved organizing a series of conferences designed to make the case for integration and to engage the white mainstream medical organizations in accomplishing it. As Cobb editorialized before the first conference convened:

The Imhotep National Conference on Hospital Integration offers
a golden opportunity to make progress in a voluntary way upon a
problem which has always been a pressing concern of the Negro

patient and physician. No responsible person associated with hospitals or the healing profession could deny that the problem has vital significance for the health of the nation as a whole and for the principles of human justice. . . ."Imhotep" means "he who cometh in peace." The sponsoring organizations, the most representative of their kind, come in peace. It is difficult to envision that any leaders of hospital groups would be unwilling to meet to discuss the problem. A first meeting of minds might afford only a start, but a constructive foundation for eventual solutions to be laid. Moreover a shining example would be afforded of how citizens of the United States can attack a vexing problem with amity and high purpose. (Cobb 1957)

The conference and subsequent ones, as the street fighters would have predicted, never got the reception Cobb hoped for. While the March 8–9, 1957, conference, as announced in the November 1956 *Journal of the National Medical Association* (*JNMA*) issue, was to be held at Howard University under the auspices of the medical school, this had to be changed at the last minute. The university was apparently concerned about possible retaliation by powerful southern legislators, and the medical school may also have been concerned about protecting scholarship funding for its students provided by southern states.[14] The Department of Health, Education and Welfare (HEW) also declined to play host, evidently for some of the same reasons. As a result, the conference was held at the Fifteenth Street Presbyterian Church, where Cobb and other prominent black physicians in Washington were members. Black churches had served as the base for organizing the civil rights movement in the South, and the national hospital component of that movement was no exception. None of the leaders of the national white medical and hospital organizations attended, and the conference received little attention in the mainstream white media.

Overall attendance dwindled at subsequent annual conferences. Faced with the lack of leadership support from the mainstream organizations, such as the American Medical Association and the American Hospital Association that might have helped generate support from their members, attention shifted in the subsequent conferences away from hope for the voluntary elimination of segregation to legislative and judicial remedies forcing it. Yet there had been little progress on these fronts, and, on the surface, the whole initiative appeared destined for failure. As one of the organizers observed: "The attendance wasn't that great and we didn't get any representation from the major organizations."[15] The Brahmin rebels pressed on.

CHARLES WATTS, MD

Charles Watts, the consummate Brahmin diplomat, worked closely with Cobb in pressing forward. He was a student of Charles Drew, sent ahead on Drew's fateful trip in 1950 to find lodging in Atlanta.[16] Education had long had a priority in Watts's family. Both Dr. Watts's parents had attended Atlanta University (then a normal school). His mother completed her degree, but his father had to drop out to run the family store after his father died. Dr. Watts's mother was one of eleven children, and her father had been born in slavery and never went to school. He made sure, however that, all his children got educated, and nine of the eleven finished college. Failing in old age, he used to refer to his grandchildren by the colleges they attended when he could no longer remember their names. "Hey you, Talladega, Hampton, he would say."[17]

During his senior year at Morehouse in 1938, Watts traveled to the University of Georgia to be interviewed as an applicant for medical school. It was a pro forma interview since the University of Georgia medical school didn't accept blacks. The NAACP was interested in using Watts as a test case for subsequent legal action. His travel to the Augusta campus was paid for by and he was the house guest of the president of Pilgrim Life Insurance (an insurance company set up to serve blacks since white life insurance companies wouldn't insure blacks and a business niche that produced many of the first black millionaires). His family background surprised the medical school professor who interviewed him. He told Watts he was the first Negro he had ever met whose parents had both attended college. His application was rejected, but, possibly in response to the pending legal action, the State of Georgia started providing Howard Medical School scholarships to black residents of Georgia.

Between graduation and enrolling in medical school at Howard the following year, in 1940, Watts had the opportunity to learn how black hospital care worked in the North. He assisted his uncle, a physician who owned a hospital in Detroit. The implicit understanding was that in Wayne County, the public facility, Detroit Receiving Hospital, was reserved to meet the needs of the white indigent, and the city of Detroit would provide support for private black hospitals to care for the black indigent so that a newer, larger public facility would not need to be constructed. "It was a terrible system," Watts said. "They couldn't maintain standards. Physicians could bring in patients for everything. There was one fellow, a very dapper fashionable fellow who liked to take tonsils out. That was when we thought every child had to have their tonsils out. Whenever, he did several tonsillectomies in the morning, we'd keep the room warm because we knew they would be back that night to stop the bleeding" (Watts 1996).

He had met his wife, Constance, in Atlanta, while he was still a student at Morehouse. Watts had been asked through family friends to entertain her and her sister during their wait to catch another train to Durham on her trip home from Talladega. Friends of the parents drove them over to Morehouse and knew they would be in good company for the day. They refused to have them sit in the filthy colored waiting room in Atlanta for five hours. Dr. Watts didn't see Constance again until he was best man at her sister's wedding in Durham. "By then she was 19 and I couldn't take my eyes off her. Three years later we were married."[18] The Merricks, as far as both black and white Durham was concerned, were aristocracy. John H. Merrick, Constance's paternal grandfather, born in slavery, had helped establish the North Carolina Mutual Insurance Company. Dr. Aaron McDuffie Moore, Constance's maternal grandfather, was a friend of John Merrick and also a cofounder of the insurance company. North Carolina Mutual is the oldest and largest black-owned insurance company in the nation. It grew and prospered, winning praise from visitors Booker T. Washington and W. E. B. DuBois and helping to make Durham known as the "Black Wall Street of America" (Weare 1993, 21). Watts would later serve as the company's medical director and as a board member.

Dr. Watts completed a surgical residency at Freedman's Hospital under Charles Drew. "There weren't many options in 1950 for persons so trained. . . . In Atlanta, there wasn't any place but a 35 bed cottage hospital where I could practice. Grady was a free hospital and I couldn't practice at any of the others and most wouldn't accept my patients."[19] Lincoln Hospital in Durham was one of the few hospitals in the country where an African American surgeon could practice, and Dr. Watts began his surgical practice there.[20] He subsequently became the first black board-certified surgeon to practice in North Carolina.

The combination of his expertise as a surgeon, his social credentials, and his warmth and human insight soon propelled him into a leadership role in negotiating across the racial medical and hospital divide in North Carolina. He became chief of surgery at Lincoln and then president of the Old North State Medical Society (ONSMS), one of the strongest state affiliates of the National Medical Association, in 1958. The Medical Society of North Carolina (MSNC) controlled appointments to the state examining board and access to continuing medical education. After joint deliberations, the MSNC offered to provide "scientific" membership to black physicians as long as they didn't have a vote and didn't attend their social functions. Not surprisingly, the ONSMS members felt this was insulting and voted not only not to accept such membership but to punish any of their members that did.

The MSNC hadn't thought any of this through far enough. It regularly had its annual meetings at Pinehurst, a world-class golf and luxury resort and that helped assure a well-attended annual meeting. In the 1950s the annual meeting at Pinehurst had been the highlight of the society's year. The general members and the wives auxiliary, in addition to the House of Delegates, joined in the festivities. The formal banquet in the main dining room of the Carolina Hotel was the highlight of the annual meeting. After MSNC decided to allow participation of blacks in the "scientific sessions," Pinehurst threw them out. "They said, we don't want any black folks down here, no Jews and no dogs or something to that effect," Dr. Watts observed, later finding humor in the slight.[21] Thus, in 1956 MSNC had to move its meetings to hotels in Asheville, lacking in any accommodations for golfers. Attendance at the subsequent annual meetings dropped by almost half. "Here they were, no blacks were attending and they were losing membership."[22]

Some of the white physicians were irritated with the black physician intransigence. They had given up the preferred home of their annual meeting to accommodate them, and the black physicians were snubbing them. On December 9, 1962, a delegation from the ONSMS headed by Dr. Watts met with the executive committee of the MSNC. When Watts's group entered and surveyed the room, "It looked like a lynching party. There were about fifty of them and I was not happy about being there." Watts tried to take cues from how Kennedy had handled the confrontation over the Cuban missile crisis about a month earlier. "We didn't want it to become a knock down and drag out fight. . . . We wanted to try to keep the negotiation on track, just as Kennedy had done." Watts told them he had full sympathy for the difficulties they were going through and was sure that with mutual respect they could all work out the changes that were necessary."[23]

Finally in May 1965 the MSNC, at an emotional session of the House of Delegates, voted to end all racial distinctions in membership. One upset member argued that "this action will do only one thing, allow Negroes to come to our dinners and dance with our women" (qtd. in Smith 1999, 73). Another accused the ONSMS of having "taken a stand on the Medicare legislation that was diametrically opposed to the stand of the AMA and this society" (qtd. in Smith 1999, 73). Neither argument held sway. The motion passed by the necessary two-thirds margin. By 1966, the Pinehurst Resort was begging them to come back, which they did in 1967, and Dr. Watts was warmly greeted at a convention dinner in the Carolina Hotel several years later by some of the retired officers of the MSNC who had participated in the earlier negotiations between the two medical societies. Pinehurst had all the ambiance of a luxurious southern plantation and used pictures of black caddies on its promotional materials as a symbol of the solicitous service its white customers would receive (just as Pullman had advertised its porters). In 1966 Pinehurst made a hard-nosed business decision. If they wanted to stay in the profitable business of hosting professional conferences, they had to bite the bullet and integrate.[24]

In November 1961 Dr. Watts entered the mainstream of Cobb's campaign to desegregate the nation's hospitals. Watts, Eaton, and Armstrong, representing ONSMS, flew to Washington to meet with HEW officials. They prodded them to address the Hill-Burton "assurance" anomaly. The 1946 Hill-Burton Act, which provided federal funding for hospital construction, required "assurances" from all applicants that the new facility would be available to all persons residing in the area without discrimination on account of race, creed, or color. While the act included an exception to this requirement in localities where "separate health facilities were planned for separate population groups," it required that the services be of like quality for each group (the separate but equal exception). The attorney general's office had previously declined to offer an opinion on the provision. Their meeting with the HEW officials was discouraging. The "assurances" of non-discrimination on the part of applicants for these funds "had never been questioned and there was no procedure for checking on the validity of the 'assurances,' nor was there any authorized course of action in a case of violations. . . . It did not appear that the Department considered it its province to know what went on in hospitals after grants had been made nor was it anxious to become involved in this area" (Cobb 1962, 259).

Dr. Armstrong, whose own son had been harmed at birth because the local white hospital had refused his wife admission for a C-section, however, got a reminder of the importance of their mission to Washington. On their arrival at National Airport, they managed to flag down a cab. After they climbed in, the black female cab driver turned around and smiled,

> "How you, Dr. Armstrong!"
> "Sugar, you know me?" Armstrong answered in surprise.
> "Yeah," the cabby answered. "I'm from Rocky Mount. You delivered me."[25]

Dr. Watts, however, had apparently been successful in engineering the quiet desegregation of the University of North Carolina Medical Center. The growth in federal funding of medical research put university medical centers in southern Jim Crow states in an awkward bind. The solution for many was to integrate but not tell anybody about it. This was apparently the case of the University of North Carolina Hospital System, according to Dr. Watts.

> We filed a suit against the University of North Carolina when I was President of the Old North State Medical Society (ONSMS). We got a student at A&T and two others admitted to the psychiatric unit at UNC. A state senator over the weekend had gotten drunk, had the DTs and was admitted to the desegregated unit. When he woke up he demanded that the hospital get them out. So the University told them they would have to leave. Two had to be sent to West Virginia for care. The state Civil Rights Commission was having a hearing in 1961. I represented the ONSMS at the hearing and I described the situation. The head UNC psychiatrist said it

had nothing to do with race, they had just found that they couldn't treat black and white patients in the same setting. I said, "Well, we're going to let the courts decide." The Chairman of the Commission called me after the meeting. He asked if I thought it would be satisfactory for ONSMS to withdraw the complaint, if the medical center just quietly integrated. He said it would hurt the University and hurt them in getting grants if we made a big public to do about it or published the fact that we had made the University change its policies. I said, we're not out to hurt the University, and it will cost us more in legal fees. If you send me a letter to that effect, I will present it to my committee. That's what they did; they sent us a letter saying that racial discrimination would no longer be allowed in the University Hospital System. They didn't relate it to our suit at all. Floyd McKissick was our lawyer. He advised us to accept it and keep the University Hospital System under observation. We filed the letter. If anybody came up with a complaint, we could trot it out. I think it cost us $200 to integrate the whole hospital system. This took place in 1962. Our purpose was to get change, not to stir up controversy.[26]

Dr. Watts's quiet negotiations were beginning to bear fruit. Indeed, Reginald Hawkins's own successes as a more confrontational street fighter in integrating Charlotte Memorial Hospital owed much to Watts's behind-the-scenes efforts. It was becoming clear that a combination of the Brown precedent and the power of the federal purse could, with sustained pressure, eliminate the most visible forms of segregation in publicly operated hospitals as well as medical school facilities. The vast majority of hospitals, however, were private voluntary ones with no connection to medical schools. As such, they remained impenetrable fortresses.

GEORGE SIMKINS JR., DDS

On December 7, 1955, six days after Rosa Parks refused to give up her seat to a white man on a Montgomery, Alabama, bus, Dr. Simkins decided to play golf. Simkins, whose father, George Simkins Sr., was also a dentist in Greensboro, had returned after completing his undergraduate degree at Talladega College and a dental degree at Meharry. He didn't have office hours Wednesday afternoons, so he corralled five of his old high school buddies and headed off to the Gillespie Park Golf Course. He had done some thinking over the previous few days, and the golf excursion was more than just a break from his practice routine. Gillespie was a white-only golf course constructed on city land as part of a WPA project in the 1930s but leased to a private group for $1 a year. (A colored golf course had also been contemplated, but it remained an overgrown patch of weeds next to the city's sewage treatment plant.) The six plunked down their greens fees and proceeded to tee off.

> We got to about the fifth or sixth hole and the pro came out. He wasn't there when we stopped by the clubhouse. He called us everything under the sun and told us we better get off or something was going to happen to us. I had a club in my hand for protection. He said, "Why are you out here?" I said, "I'm out here for a cause." "What kind of G-damn cause?" he asked. "The cause of democracy!" I answered. That statement made him all red and he was just mad. The fellow was cursing and cursing.[27]

Simkins never backed down. They were jailed, his father posted the bond, and they appealed. The judge on the appeal to state court set the tone: "If you had come out on my place I would have probably got my shotgun. I'm going to give you all thirty days in jail. Take them away, sheriff." That judge had also taken Simkins aside and berated him for "playing with guys that didn't have the same educational level, one was a chauffeur, one was a cab driver, one was a barber and so forth. He was trying to divide us."[28] In the meantime they had gone to federal court and gotten a judgment that they had the right to do what they did, and the golf course was given three weeks to integrate. The club house "mysteriously" burned down two days before the deadline, and the fire marshal condemned the whole property. No one, black or white, could play golf there for seven years until it was finally opened on an integrated basis. Unlike the public buses that middle-class white professionals didn't use, the closing of the golf course got their attention. It was not the only golf course desegregation case handled by the NAACP Legal Defense Fund for health professionals, and it struggled with trying to make sense out of investing resources in something that didn't seem to be such a civil rights priority. It was, however, a group that provided a substantial portion of their funding and whose interests could not be ignored.

Simkins soon became president of the Greensboro branch of the NAACP and a major force in its desegregation efforts. Greensboro had more of a history as a company town, rather than one seeking the relocation of new businesses as was the case of Charlotte. Its white leadership, as a consequence, was more intransigent on civil rights matters. Just as the golf course, the city swimming pool was closed rather than be forced to integrate. Most remember Greensboro for the A&T student lunch counter sit-in that began in the downtown Woolworth's and spread rapidly across the country. Simkins had met with its leaders and helped guide their plan.

A combination of events, however, propelled Simkins into the center of the hospital desegregation struggle. His efforts, more than those of any other individual, propelled an implausible chain reaction of events that would transform health care in the United States.

Typical of larger communities in North Carolina, Greensboro had a meticulously segregated hospital system. Moses Cone, the largest, best-endowed hospital was for most purposes white only. It provided segregated accommodations but only to black patients for whose conditions L. Richardson, the city's black hospital, didn't have the equipment to treat. Another hospital, Wesley Long, accepted only white admissions. All three of Greensboro's hospitals were private not-for-profit ones, and all had received Hill-Burton funds for hospital construction. Most medical professionals, both black and white, felt that this was a perfectly reasonable set of arrangements. Moses Cone felt, if a little patronizingly, protective of L. Richardson Hospital. Direct competition with Richardson, the weaker partner, might force its closing. Black doctors at least had privileges at Richardson. It was not clear whether they could all get privileges at Moses Cone or Wesley Long if they became integrated, or how restrictive those privileges might be.

The problem, however, as Simkins concluded, was that separate was never going to be equal. He turned to Thurgood Marshall and Jack Greenberg, from whom he had sought help with the federal court case involving the Gillespie Park Golf Course.

A patient came into my office, a young A&T student. His jaw was swollen with an abscessed third molar. He had a temperature of

103. I said, "Young man, you need to be hospitalized." The hospital (L. Richardson) was one block from my office. I called up there to get him a room. They said, "I'm sorry doc, we've got a waiting list of two or three weeks before you can get a bed." They actually had patients in the hallways. You had to walk a narrow path through the corridors because the patient beds were in the hallways. I called Moses Cone, and they had rooms over there, but they wouldn't take him. I called Wesley Long and the same thing. Then I called Jack Greenberg, who had taken Thurgood Marshall's place. I said, "We got to really do something about these hospitals down here. It's a disgrace, a person could be dying." He said, "George, if you can get the black doctors organized and do some research and find out how much Hill-Burton funds have gone into building those hospitals, I'll take the case." I got busy and got the young doctors I knew I could get signed on to be plaintiffs. When the older docs saw the names, some of them signed and some didn't. I got each of them to put up fifty bucks for attorney fees. We lost the case in Middle District Court and appealed.[29]

It was through Dr. Simkins's efforts, however, in bringing this case, that Dr. Cobb finally got the break he had been fighting for. As the seventh and final Imhotep Conference convened on May 25, 1963, Cobb presented the dwindling attendees with a surprise telegram.

> I am sure you are aware that the Attorney General has intervened in a federal court case, arguing that the clause sanctioning segregation in the Hill-Burton Act is unconstitutional.
> I am hopeful, as I know you are, that this action will speed the day when all will recognize that we cannot afford to squander our resources on the practice of racial discrimination and that the availability of hospital services will not depend on the race, color or creed of the patient.
> I wish you a successful conference.
> John F. Kennedy. (Kennedy 1962, 501)

The street fighters and the Brahmin rebels now had a new team member whose backbone had yet to be tested.

3

Better Part of Valor

Kennedy's telegram to Cobb marked a watershed event. However reluctantly, based on their cold calculations of what was politically possible, Presidents Kennedy and then Johnson would follow the lead of the medical activists. Step by step, the activists drew them into using the untested power of federal dollars to force radical change in some of the most powerful institutions in the country.

Kennedy's "Mandate"

The deck is, of course, stacked toward giving importance to the "decisions" of presidents rather than the diffuse effect of social movements on political will. Every word of a president is monitored and every action analyzed. From Harry Truman onward, presidential libraries have functioned as endowed public relations agents, preserving presidents' words and actions, promoting their timeless importance on the world stage. For example, even before the release of the 2015 film *Selma*, on the 1965 march for voting rights, editorials appeared in *Politico* by the director of the Johnson Library and in the *Washington Post* by presidential aide Joseph Califano objecting to the film's portrayal of Lyndon Johnson, both using the resources of the library to make their case (Undergrove 2014; Califano 2014).

The debate about the contributions of Presidents Kennedy and Johnson to the civil rights reforms of the 1960s continues. Certainly both were skillful role players. Yet presidents get both more credit and more blame than they deserve. More often than not, they are swept along by larger events beyond their control. In no case was this truer than with the Kennedy and Johnson administrations. They were, I will argue, but bit players in that larger drama. Consider the "opening act" that propelled Kennedy's election.[1]

Jailed for participating in a student-organized demonstration against segregated stores in Atlanta, Martin Luther King faced retaliation. While the local and state legal system released the student demonstrators, they sentenced King on a trumped-up traffic misdemeanor charge to four months hard labor on a prison road gang, transferred him to a rural state prison, and denied bail.

Concerned about a brutal sentence that could cost him his life, Coretta King and civil rights leaders pressed the Kennedy and Nixon campaigns in the last week of a tightly contested election to intervene. Black voters generally viewed Nixon and the Republican Party more favorably than Kennedy and the Democrats, but the Nixon campaign chose to ignore these appeals. At the same time, Kennedy's campaign strategists were desperate to avoid appearing to side with the civil rights activists, certain that would cost Kennedy the loss of the southern states, the so-called solid South, and the election.

Responding to the pleas of Harris Wofford, the campaign's liaison with the civil rights movement, Sargent Shriver went behind the backs of the campaign's chief strategists and approached Kennedy, while he was resting in private, exhausted from nonstop campaigning in the Chicago area. He urged Kennedy to just make a personal courtesy call to Mrs. King. Kennedy reluctantly agreed. He spoke briefly on the phone to her, "I know this must be very hard for you. I understand you are expecting a baby, and I just wanted you to know that I was thinking about you and Dr. King. If there is anything I can do to help, please feel free to call me" (qtd. in Branch 1988, 362). Enraged, Robert Kennedy, his brother's campaign manager, lashed out, "You bomb throwers have lost the whole campaign!" (qtd. in Branch 1988, 364).

While the call and the subsequent change of heart and intervention by Robert Kennedy that got King out on bail were downplayed and caused only a brief ripple in the mainstream media, it changed the outcome of the election. Wofford and Shriver made arrangements for the distribution of "The Blue Bomb," two million leaflets to black churches the Sunday before the election. It described the call to Coretta King and touched a chord in the black community long fragmented by party loyalties. Kennedy went on to win the election by a popular margin of 49.7 percent to Nixon's 49.5 percent. Without the black vote, Nixon would have won 52 percent of the popular vote, carried Illinois and Michigan, and won the election. In the 1956 election blacks had voted 60 percent for Eisenhower. In 1960, 70 percent of blacks voted for Kennedy. An

American president, for the first time, owed his election to the black vote. Kennedy, however, recognizing his narrow margin of victory and the certain defeat any civil rights legislation would face, avoided taking promised legislative action for more than two years.

Executive Inaction

Kennedy's ability to acknowledge his electoral debt through executive action was no more promising. True, Truman had desegregated the military and federal agencies by executive order. However, using an executive order to bar discrimination in state and local governments and private agencies receiving federal support was without precedent. Indeed, Harlem congressman Adam Clayton Powell (D, NY) had repeatedly hit a brick wall, submitting amendments to almost every bill involving federal funding since the late 1940s that were routinely rejected. No laws passed in the twentieth century prohibited the use of federal funds to support segregation, and one, the Hill-Burton Act of 1946, explicitly permitted it. Congressional intent seemed clear, and any effort of Kennedy's to block the use of federal funds for such purposes would be challenged.

The Civil Rights Leadership Council, an umbrella organization representing most of the civil rights groups, launched its own challenge, submitting a report to the new administration in August 1961. While acknowledging the initiation of some positive steps, the report observed that these actions were "dwarfed, and, in fact nullified, by the massive involvement of the federal government in programs and activities that make it a silent but nonetheless full partner in the perpetuation of discriminatory practices" (Wilkins and Aronson 1961, 2). The numbers in the document were the most telling part of the argument. A state-by-state table listed the ratio of federal taxes paid to federal dollars received. The average for eleven southern states was less than .5 and the average for eleven northern states was more than 1.5. In other words, the federal government served as the vehicle for subsidizing discriminatory practices in southern states with the money received from the taxpayers of northern states, where such practices were prohibited.[2]

Harris Wofford, assigned as Kennedy's special assistant for civil rights, struggled in Kennedy's first year in office to find a way that would satisfy its debt to its black constituency and the demands of the civil rights groups. An interagency subcabinet task force set up by Wofford had come up with few answers, and even these had been challenged by the Department of Health, Education and Welfare (HEW) general counsel (Banta 1961). Assistant secretary of HEW James Quigley, in a memo to Wofford in November 1961, did not question the correctness of the Leadership Council's assessment but expressed concern about the disruption any sweeping executive order would impose on people dependent on benefits, including blacks. In addition, he noted that the constitutionality of such an order was dubious (Quigley 1961). None of the authorizing legislation supporting HEW programs prohibited segregation, and two, the Hill-Burton Act of 1946, supporting hospital construction, and the Morrill Land-Grant Act of 1890, providing funds for racially segregated land-grant educational institutions, specifically permitted it. Until the constitutionality of either of those two legislative precedents was successfully challenged, any such executive order was certain to fail to stop federally subsidized segregation.

Desegregating the Medical School Hospitals

These restrictions did not prevent the Kennedy administration from playing a discrete chess game with recipients of federal funding, pressuring them to end segregation. The nation's medical schools were an obvious target. The growth in federal funding of medical research in the post–World War II era had transformed medical schools. The years between 1955 and 1968 were remembered as "the Golden Years" of National Institutes of Health (NIH) expansion (National Institutes of Health 2013). Not only did the federal government become the dominant source of research funding for medical schools during this period, but, more importantly, it ceded control over the distribution of those funds to the scientific community (Starr 1982, 343). As a result, research grant review committees through a combination of subtle guidance, selection, and predilections, made it clear to medical schools that they had to choose between Jim Crow practices and federal research funding. These efforts were reinforced by Assistant Secretary James Quigley and by Sherry Arnstein, who directed compliance activities, after the passage of the Civil Rights Act in 1964 (Reynolds 1997).

This put university medical centers in southern states with Jim Crow laws in an awkward bind. The solution, as illustrated in the last chapter by Dr. Watts's account of the integration of the University of North Carolina Medical Center, was to integrate but not tell anybody about it.

Dr. Charles Johnson, who would later serve as president of the NMA in 1990–1991, went to Duke in 1964 for a fellowship in endocrinology, just as the school was beginning to transition in response to federal pressures. He later described his experience:

> I was told by the Division Chief that he didn't want me going on the private side because some of the physicians were concerned about the reaction of their patients. I felt I was signed on under false pretenses. It turned out that the Division was trying to get a Biometrics Lab funded by NIH. Dr. Fine from the University of Michigan and two others were on the site visit. They questioned the endocrine fellows. We were all sitting at the table, all nine. At the end of the session, Dr. Fine asked, "Are any of you unhappy about the training you have received?" I said, "Yes I am. I have been told that I can't rotate on the private side because of my color." He said, "What did you say?" I said, "I have been told that I can't rotate on the private side because of my color." He said, "Well, we'll see about that!" The other fellows came to my support. I hadn't known what they felt before. Anyways, the senior faculty and Chief of the Division followed the fellows. The first question asked the Chief of the Division was, "Why can't Dr. Johnson rotate on the private side of the hospital?" No answer. I never heard the inner working of what did and didn't get said after that but I'm certain a lot of money got tied up in the discussion. Ed Horton who was doing research related to transplanting diabetics and who is now at Harvard called me and said, "I think you better stay away from here until the dust settles." Finally, the Chief met with me. He had lost his voice by the way, he could not talk for several days—race relations is always a touchy question and if it's the first question it creates a state of shock. The man really lost his voice. He says, "Dr. Johnson, do you really want to rotate on the private service?" . . . I rotated. Clearly they accepted the money and me too. Otherwise, they would have lost a large sum of government money. It wasn't that they wanted me so bad, they wanted the money more. They needed a big stick waved over their heads."[3]

Even the well-funded state enforcer of segregation, the Mississippi Sovereignty Commission, which operated out of the governor's office, had to concede in a chess game that began to be played out in the 1960s over the future of the University of Mississippi Medical Center in Jackson (Smith 2005, 256–60).[4] Dr. Robert Marston, former Rhodes Scholar, who later served as NIH director, was director and dean of the University of Mississippi Medical Center at this time. He and others recruited apparently had little sympathy with the Sovereignty Commission's mission. They were concerned about building the reputation of the medical school and hospital. Following its usual procedures, the commission sent detectives to investigate complaints. A nurse in 1960 had complained that a personnel director and nurses in charge were all from the North and that these nurses had compelled white nurses to work on "colored" floors and black nurses to work on white floors, and that the elevator operators were now all black and were allowing black visitors to ride the same elevators as white visitors. Another informant complained that one of the doctors at the center had been lecturing at medical schools around the world and that some of the students from these schools who had visited the medical center in Jackson were black. In 1964, a Sovereignty Commission detective reported that segregation at the medical center was on the verge of collapse. The parking lots were integrated, and the white and colored patients used the same waiting room in the X-ray department. "Since there is only one cobalt machine and all the X-rays are adjacent to the waiting room. I do not know how the hospital authorities can remedy this congestion of the mixing of Negroes and Whites, except through expansion" (Smith 2005, 257). The obstetrics and pediatric services were a particular source of concern to the investigator. There was one labor room with eight beds used for both black and white women, and they all used the same four delivery rooms. After their deliveries, the black mothers were placed on a separate floor, but their babies remained on the same floor in a segregated nursery next to the nursery for white babies and near where the white mothers were placed. On the pediatric floor, children of both races shared a common area and playroom. The black and white patients were not supposed to use the playroom at the same time, although staff admitted that this rule was seldom enforced. The investigator aptly summarized the dilemma the Medical Center posed for the protection of Mississippi's "sovereignty."

The University Hospital is a very fine institution and composed
of some of the best doctors and instructors in the Nation and is a
credit to the State of Mississippi. Mississippi people are proud of the
University Hospital, but there are no doubts in my mind but that
improvements can be brought about at the University to improve on
the creeping integration which is in evidence out there. I am sure it
will cost the state extra money, but Mississippi should by all means
provide the extra cash needed to maintain proper segregation at
University Hospital. (qtd. in Smith 2005, 258)

In other words, if the state was really committed to preserving
segregation, it should pay for it. In early 1964, the US Army Medical
Research and Development Commission advised the University that
it would have to comply with the federal executive orders banning segregation. Dean Marston made clear to the director of the Sovereignty
Commission that this would be just the beginning of similar compliance orders from other federal agencies that would involve the loss of at
least 5.3 million dollars in federal support. In its report to the governor
the commission outlined the options that might be considered.

It is inconceivable at this time that the State Legislature would be
in a position to supplement the appropriations for the Medical
Center and replace the federal funds flowing to the Center or in the
available future. . . . In a way this leaves us in a somewhat untenable
position. We can yield and assure continuance of the funds, which
would be against our policies, we could advise the Army [that] we
cannot comply with the request and lose the army research grant;
we could continue the present segregated facility policies and take
the chance that many months or years would transpire before each
of the various agencies served similar notice about the facilities;
or we could write off all the federal funds for the Medical Center
and seek some method of replacing these funds with either state or
private money or both. (qtd. in Smith 2005, 259)

The state of Mississippi opted to take the money. The Sovereignty Commission suggested some convoluted ways to eliminate visible symbols
of segregation while possibly preserving "voluntary" segregation. These
suggestions appear to have been ignored by the medical center.

Southern medical schools desegregated in stages, picking the safest targets first. The first units to be desegregated were the ones most insulated from public scrutiny—newly created intensive care units. These units began to be set up in medical school hospitals in the early 1960s in order to provide better care for the critically ill patients. At the University of North Carolina Medical Center, an early special care unit had one room with three beds and one with four. Nurses were supposed to move black patients to keep the races separate. This meant extra work for the nurses and would sometimes compromise care. Cookie Wilson, a nurse who had a long career at the medical center later recalled in 2002, "I was just a rotating staff nurse at the time, but I got tired of that. It was ridiculous. So, I did not move them. I integrated the unit." No family complaints and no hospital reprimand followed. "Nobody opened their mouth" (Broom 2002).

Dr. Chris Hansen, a white physician in Mississippi who served on a civil rights group hospital compliance committee, offered a similar story about the University of Mississippi Medical Center. Hansen met with its director, Dr. Robert Marston. Marston assured him that the medical center was making slow but steady progress. He said, "I know it is slow, but I want to tell you as a measure of our good faith that we have our first integrated ward and I'm going to take you up and show it to you" (qtd. in Geiger 2013). He took them upstairs and showed them, and there, indeed, was a four-bed male ward with four patients: two African Americans, a white man and a Native American. All four of them were unconscious. They had achieved their first step at integration with four people in comas (Geiger 2013). Neither comatose ICU patients nor their families, focused on the survival of their loved one, were going to pay much attention to who was in the bed next to them. In addition, from the hospital's standpoint, the cost of creating two separate ICUs, no matter what their racial views, was hard to justify.

By the end of 1965 most of the medical school–run hospitals in the Jim Crow South were on the way toward being integrated. In most cases this had been done secretly with many denying any change in policies. While the changes had been facilitated by supportive medical school deans and university administrators, it was the threat of the loss of federal funding and the budget crisis it presented to the universities and states that silenced the segregationist opposition.

The Northern Front

The civil rights movement efforts understandably focused on the highly visible, morally repugnant symbols of the Jim Crow South such as blacks' being restricted to seats only on the back of the bus, their exclusion from lunch counters, and the separate entrances and waiting rooms they were forced to use. None of these visible symbols existed in the North. However, invisible color lines in most northern cities, reinforced by real estate practices, custom, and, when necessary, mob violence, assured almost an equivalent degree of segregation. It is easy to make the visible symbols disappear and leave less visible racial advantages unchanged. It is easier to take the moral high ground on the visible symbols, much harder for invisible boundaries that directly affect one's pocketbook and life chances. This was the northern problem, which was no better illustrated than by the hospitals in the city of Chicago.

As described in the last chapter, it had taken a ten-year struggle just to get public officials and hospital leaders to acknowledge that racial segregation existed in Chicago's hospitals. No equivalent of a George Wallace stood in the doorways, but an invisible color line, reflected in the hospital privileging process and physician admitting practices, assured almost the same degree of segregation that existed in communities in the Deep South. This invisible form of segregation was finally challenged in federal court.

On February 10, 1961, ten Chicago physicians filed suit in United States Federal District Court, Northern District of Illinois, and Eastern Division. The plaintiffs, acting on behalf of more than two hundred black physicians in Chicago, alleged that the defendants (the five medical and hospital associations representing medical staffs and hospitals in the Chicago area as well as fifty-six hospitals), in denying privileges to black doctors and services to black patients, were in violation of the Sherman Antitrust Act (Cobb 1961). At the time the suit was initiated, there were only sixteen out of a total of 226 active black physicians in Chicago who had some form of staff appointment at one of Chicago's historically white voluntary hospitals (J. Morris 1960). Seventy-two of these black physicians were eligible for specialty certification. Only eight of the seventy-eight historically white private hospitals in the area provided any black physicians with privileges. The black population was increasing in Chicago, but the number of black doctors practicing in Chicago was declining, financially squeezed out of the Chicago medical market. As a result, their patients with Blue Cross insurance, in spite of sales material assuring access to enrollees to any participating hospitals, were forced to rely on the already overcrowded public hospitals. Since the public hospitals were "non-participating" in the Blue Cross plan, they were provided with much lower payments. Black Blue Cross subscribers thus subsidized lower premiums for white subscribers and higher profits for the Blue Cross plan. Since the Blue Cross payments to the public hospitals did not cover the full cost of care, as they did for the private hospitals, these arrangements also added to the costs borne by taxpayers. In most southern states, the visible color line under the Hill-Burton separate but equal provisions had tended to narrow the gap in the number of hospital beds available to blacks as compared to whites (Thomas 2011, 207). Chicago, with its invisible color line, the plaintiffs argued, offered whites four hospital beds per one thousand, and blacks only .65 beds per one thousand (R. Morris 1960, 195).

Arguing along lines that had been successfully used previously for physicians excluded from hospital privileges because of participating in managed care plans, the plaintiffs demanded relief and treble damages. The American Medical Association and its local constituent societies had waged a long war against early managed care plans that they considered "socialized" medicine and an unethical form of medical practice (Starr 1982, 302–6). They worked to block them as competitors by preventing physicians working with them from getting hospital privileges. In a key case used by the plaintiffs in the Chicago suit, the AMA and its District of Columbia affiliate had been convicted of conspiring to violate the Sherman Antitrust Act by blocking hospital privileges for physicians participating in Group Health, a cooperative plan set up by federal employees, and the decision was upheld by the Supreme Court (*American Medical Association v. United States* 317 US 519 (1943). Organized medicine's battle against managed care continued into the 1970s. The AMA and its constituent societies eventually accommodated to such arrangements, and managed care became part of the medical mainstream. In an ironic twist, by 2000 the National Medical Association was protesting discrimination and exclusion of minorities from participation in such plans (Shervington 2000).

The Chicago antitrust suit got everyone's attention. Treble the foregone lifetime earnings of two hundred physicians would have amounted to billions and, in the event that such an award had been made, would have bankrupted all the voluntary hospitals in Chicago.

If the plaintiffs had just argued on moral grounds that they and their patients had been discriminated against because of their race, the best that could have been achieved was modest embarrassment for the defendants and a promise to do better in the future. Cobb, understandably, celebrated the event in his Integration Battlefront column, arguing that the physicians involved in the suit "merit the gratitude and appreciation of Negro physicians everywhere for blowing the first legal blast of the trumpet against the racial walls of Jericho around the hospitals in Chicago. . . . It is to be hoped that Court action in this present case will send them tumblin' down" (Cobb 1961, 199). Many of the black professional colleagues of the plaintiffs, however, were not as appreciative. As Arthur Falls, one of the plaintiffs, later observed: "It was considered a very dangerous thing by many of our colleagues. We started with ten physicians and then two dropped out. Actually some members of the staff at Provident (the black hospital in Chicago) stopped speaking to us" (Falls 1988). Responding to the attention, the Chicago City Council passed an ordinance the following year forbidding racial discrimination in the appointment and employment of physicians, imposing a fine of between $100 and $200 a day.

The plaintiffs in the suit, however, faced bitter disappointment through the adroit handling by the city's white establishment. The city ordinance never resulted in any fines, and the suit was sidetracked. The judge chose to appoint a commission to work out a settlement rather than take the antitrust case to trial. The commission, with one representative from the plaintiffs' side, one from the defendants,' and a court-appointed chair, were assigned responsibility to hear individual complaints related to hospital privilege decisions and work out a settlement. Not surprisingly, according to Quentin Young, no complaints were forthcoming. "No one wanted to bring a complaint. On a hospital staff where survival depends on others whether in terms of referrals and medical staff assignments, no one is going to thrive who has forced their entry to a staff where the majority opposed their membership. Black doctors are just as much careerist as white doctors and they're just not going to commit the equivalent of professional suicide."[5]

In the meantime Mayor Richard Daly, possibly under pressure from the judge embarrassed by the result of his decision, created his own commission. Its official title was the Special Committee on Staff Appointment for Negro Physicians of the Chicago Commission on Human Relations, but as Quentin Young later observed it was known by the participants as "Mayor Daly's Commission." All the key medical power brokers in the city were represented. "He appointed a distinguished Cook County circuit court justice to chair it, and the heads of the Hospital Council, Chicago Archdiocese, Medical Society and the City's major hospitals." They also appointed Dr. Quentin Young and Dr. "Phi" Phillips, a black surgeon who had worked with the Committee to End Discrimination in Chicago Medical Institutions. As Dr. Young later explained:

> We were placed on the Commission so we could witness the transactions. If I ever write a book, I would call this chapter *The Meat Market*. These people would sit down and barter about who and with what credentials they were willing to accept on their staff. By the end you could actually say any black physician that wanted an appointment on the staff of a "predominantly white hospital" had one. It may not have been their first choice or near their practice but they had an appointment. About half the black docs, the older ones that had been subjected to all the insults of the segregated system for too long, weren't interested but the younger ones, particularly the surgeons happily accepted it. It was a rather amazing city-wide resolution of something that typically happened elsewhere in bits and pieces in other cities as a result of court suits related to individual hospitals. What the Mayor Daly's Commission actually did, since there weren't enough black physicians to make a real difference in admission patterns was to give white staff members permission to admit their black patients rather than admitting them only to Cook and Provident.[6]

As this account illustrates, the desegregation of hospitals in northern cities that had invisible color lines followed a more tortuous path and, in many ways, was more incomplete than what eventually happened in the South, where there was nothing subtle about the color lines. Yet in both the North and the South successful desegregation hinged more on money than moral persuasion. The Kennedy administration, coming to this realization, tied their hopes to lending its support to the case brought by Dr. George Simkins in Greensboro, North Carolina.

The Major Campaign: *Simkins v. Moses Cone*

The low-profile desegregation of southern medical schools and skir-mishes in some northern cities were just a prelude to the major cam-paign. The vast majority of hospitals in the nation were left unchanged. They didn't receive federal training and research funds and didn't have a Mayor Daly who could press for a cumbersome partial solution to medical staff segregation. Almost all hospitals, however, had received Hill-Burton funding for construction. Dr. Simkins did his homework as requested by the Legal Defense Fund. Both Moses Cone Hospital and Wesley Long Hospital had relied on substantial Hill-Burton fund-ing for expansions. The funds required compliance with federal and state regulations including demonstration that the projects fit within a state plan in terms of bed needs. The case, the Legal Defense Fund attorneys felt, hinged on demonstrating that a governmental function was being carried out by these "private" hospitals and thus their "sepa-rate but equal" arrangements were unconstitutional. If this argument prevailed, it would have profound implications.

Any federal district court faced with a suit challenging the con-stitutionality of an act of Congress is required to notify the attorney general and permit the Justice Department to intervene to provide evidence of its constitutionality (US Code, section 2403). In the *Sim-kins* case, that notification produced an "Aha!" moment in Attorney General Robert Kennedy's office. The suit was a gift, a piece to the puzzle that offered an elegant way out of the Kennedy administration's civil rights dilemma. No constitutionally questionable and politically suicidal executive order would be necessary. All that would be needed was a little low-profile support by the executive branch to nudge the federal courts to the right decision. The administration then, in insist-ing on nondiscrimination requirements for *any* federal funds flowing to state, local, and private agencies, would, arguably, only be comply-ing with the law of the land as established by the federal courts. Po-litically it seemed almost risk-free. Presidents stand for reelection but federal judges don't.

The suit was filed in federal district court in February 1962. Assis-tant Attorney General Burke Marshall requested permission to inter-vene, not as would typically be the case to defend the constitutionality of a federal law, but on behalf of the plaintiffs. Jack Greenberg and Mi-chael Melzer, the Legal Defense Fund attorneys, were surprised and delighted to have the support. The Moses Cone Hospital and Wesley Long Hospital legal team were outraged. One of defendants' lawyers protested to the local paper:

> The intervention sought by the United States in this case is apparently without precedent. The defendants have not been able to find any case in which the Attorney General of the United States has ever sought to intervene in order to attack—rather than defend the constitutionality of an Act of Congress; and the Attorney General— through his representatives at the hearing before this court on May 14, 1962—conceded that he had also not found any such a case. . . . That even if the action of the Attorney General in this case does not directly flout congressional mandate, it is certainly calculated to disappoint congressional expectation: and that is clearly contrary to the purpose of and the tradition under Section 2403. (*Greensboro Daily News* 1962, 1)

The case now began to take on an importance for private hospitals that the *Brown* case had for public schools. The federal district court judge ruled in favor of the defendants and dismissed the case in December 1962. The plaintiffs appealed and argued the case before the Fourth Circuit Court of Appeals in April 1963. The Greensboro hospitals were not an isolated aberration. At least eighty-nine all-black or all-white "separate but equal" hospitals had been built with Hill-Burton funds. In November 1963 the court ruled in favor of the appellants. The defendants appealed to the Supreme Court, and the stakes got even higher. On March 2, 1964, the Supreme Court, in an unusually expedited decision, refused to review the *Simkins* case and allowed the Fourth Circuit Court of Appeals decision on the unconstitutionality of the Hill-Burton separate but equal provision to stand.

Title VI and the Civil Rights Bill

Kennedy's Civil Rights Bill shadowed through Congress; the *Simkins* case through the courts. In May 1963 Bull Connor had turned high-pressure fire hoses and police dogs on children protesting segregated public accommodations in Birmingham. On June 11, 1963, George Wallace, in a carefully orchestrated performance, blocked the enrollment of two black students to the University of Alabama. That evening on national television, Kennedy introduced his promised but long-delayed Civil Rights Bill. Later that same evening, as if in response to Kennedy's address, Medgar Evers, field secretary for the Mississippi NAACP, was assassinated in his driveway in Jackson, Mississippi. The most controversial section of Kennedy's bill, Title VI, dealt not with more morally repugnant visible symbols of Jim Crow but with the money. It reflected the same thinking that had propelled the *Simkins* case. In his televised message, Kennedy tried to understate its significance.

> Simple justice requires that public funds, to which all taxpayers of all races contribute, not be spent in any fashion which encourages, entrenches, subsidizes or results in racial discrimination. Direct discrimination by federal, state or local governments is prohibited by the Constitution. But indirect discrimination through the use of federal funds is just as invidious; and it should not be necessary to resort to the courts to prevent each individual violation. (Kennedy 1964)

The bill, strengthened by a coalition of liberal Democrats and Republicans happy to let the president be blamed for whatever watering down would follow, found its way from the Judiciary Committee to the House Rules Committee. Its fate, in the hands of a fragile bipartisan alliance, hung by a thread. On November 22, 1963, an assassin's bullet in Dallas ended the life of its reluctant architect.

In the meantime, the Mississippi Sovereignty Commission was busy during this period organizing a well-financed campaign to defeat Kennedy's Civil Rights Bill. That campaign included all the paranoid hysteria and misinformation that shaped and continues to shape campaigns to block federal efforts to expand health insurance coverage. With the support of more recently established sovereignty commissions in Alabama and Louisiana and a $100,000 ($774,000 in current dollars) donation from a bank in New York City from an anonymous donor, they set up a lobbying office in Washington, DC, the Coordinating Committee for Fundamental American Freedom, Inc. Their mass mailings, as well as full-page ads targeting papers in states in the Midwest and West, included an attack on the Civil Rights Bill that labeled it "The Socialist Omnibus Bill of 1963." Targeting Title VI, the mailing told readers, "You should know, through this bill, you are to be struck with a $100 Billion Blackjack—almost the entire federal budget. Your tax money is to be used as a weapon against you" (Mississippi Sovereignty Commission 1964b). The bill, it claimed, would give the president the power to do anything he thought appropriate and federal agencies the power to "determine by itself what is or is not 'discrimination'—the bill itself does not define the word. . . . Six members of the House Judiciary Committee, all attorneys and all experts on this type of legislation have said: '(This) bill is not a "moderate" bill and it has not been "watered down."' It constitutes the greatest grasp of executive power conceived in the 20th Century" (Mississippi Sovereignty Commission 1964b). As Earle Johnson, the director of the Mississippi Sovereignty Commission, noted after a meeting of the Coordinating Committee in Washington in January 1964, the promotional campaign was all part of a coordinated strategy. "The overall strategy as mapped out by Senator Jim Eastland (D, MS) and other Southern senators is to keep the civil rights act as strong as possible without weakening them by amendment. It is considered likely in its present state, it is so repugnant to many senators that they will not approve cloture and the bills can be killed through filibuster" (Mississippi Sovereignty Commission 1964a).

On the other side of this legislative divide, Martin Luther King Jr. and Lyndon Baines Johnson struggled to form a fragile partnership. At 9:20 p.m. on November 25, 1963, three days after Kennedy's assassination, Johnson called King. He told him of the difficulty he faced with the Civil Rights Bill and related legislation and thanked him for the support he had offered in a statement. "I want to tell you how grateful I am for your support and how worthy I am going to try to be of all your hopes." King thanked him for this and for his "great spirit" in the difficult times they now faced. "One of the great tributes we can pay in memory of President Kennedy is to try to enact all the great progressive policies that he sought to initiate," King said (L. Johnson 1963b). Johnson assured him he was going to "support them all, do his best to get others to support them" and asked for King's help. In closing, he invited him to visit him in the White House and to bring any suggestions he had with him (L. Johnson 1963b). Just two days later, in his address to a joint session of Congress and a stunned nation, Johnson asked for their support as well. "First, no memorial oration or eulogy could more eloquently honor President Kennedy's memory than the earliest possible passage of the civil rights bill for which he fought for so long. We have talked long enough in this country about equal rights. We have talked for one hundred years or more. It is now time to write the next chapter, and to write it in the books of law" (L. Johnson 1963a, 3).

This marked the beginning of Johnson's partnership as president with the civil rights movement (Kotz 2005). Johnson met with King at the White House on December 3, 1963. Other civil rights leaders had similar sessions with the new president. All were struck by the focused, task-oriented nature of these meetings rather than the more cautious and largely passive approach taken by his predecessor. The ambition of the broad, loosely connected, grassroots, social movement that King had become the titular leader of exceeded Johnson's own. Their shared agenda encompassed civil rights, voting rights, educational access, economic development, poverty eradication, and, almost as an afterthought, health care equity. Each saw all as interrelated pieces of the same essential national transformation. Vice President Johnson's speech at Gettysburg on Memorial Day, a few months before the Kennedy assassination, to commemorate the one hundredth anniversary of the battle that marked the turning point of the Civil War, expressed urgency about this civil rights agenda that surprised many who had written him off as just another southern politician. His words captured as well as any of the better remembered ones of King the vision of that transformation.

> In this hour, it is not our respective races which are at stake—it is our nation. Let those who care for their country come forward, North and South, white and Negro, to lead the way through this moment of challenge and decision. The Negro says, "Now." Others say, "Never." The voice of responsible Americans—the voice of those who died here and the great man who spoke here—their voices say, "Together." There is no other way. Until justice is blind to color, until education is unaware of race, until opportunity is unconcerned with the color of men's skins, emancipation will be a proclamation but not a fact. To the extent that the proclamation of emancipation is not fulfilled in fact, to that extent we shall have fallen short of assuring freedom to the free." (L. Johnson 1963c)

In the five turbulent years that followed, much changed. The civil rights–driven transformation of health care was almost invisible in that larger, more public national drama. Yet, in many respects, it was the movement's most significant and lasting accomplishment.

Moses Cone Memorial Hospital and the "company town leadership" of Greensboro, North Carolina, were not in the habit of caving in to the pressure of civil rights groups or even the full force of the federal government. Cone's hospital administrators had been confidentially in regular touch with the hospitals involved in similar disputes, including the administrator at James Walker Memorial Hospital in Wilmington, North Carolina, where Hubert Eaton's group of black physicians was engaged in a legal struggle to gain privileges. The lawyers engaged in the *Cone* appeal had also exchanged correspondence with the lawyers representing Grady Memorial in Atlanta, which, lacking the defense of being a private entity, was attempting to argue that its continued segregation was justified on the basis of sound medical practice even though they were doubtful they would prevail. The lawyers representing the Moses Cone and Wesley Long hospitals had also sought support with their appeal to the Supreme Court, with amicus briefs from the AMA and AHA. These were apparently declined on technical grounds. Reflecting on the work of the firm representing them, Moses Cone's administrator reflected, "They gave it the works. We made a scrap of it."[7] The unbudgeted legal expense of more than $100,000 in current dollars, however, was a source of discomfort for the board chairman. Even at the end, when the Supreme Court had rejected their appeal, Cone's hospital executive committee had called an emergency meeting of the full board to consider the proposal that the hospital return all the Hill-Burton funds it had received, together with interest, "in order to be relieved of any obligation under the orders of the Court entered as a result of the Hospital having received Hill-Burton funds" (Moses Cone Hospital Board 1964, 1048). The full board declined to consider this option, and the hospital began the process of accommodating to the decision.

The Senate had yet to begin debate on the Civil Rights Bill, and its southern senators were not in the habit of caving in either. The option of inserting a Hill-Burton-type clause that would permit the use of federal funds under Title VI on a "separate but equal" basis as a way to circumvent a filibuster was certainly under consideration. On February 26, 1964, by a majority vote, the Senate placed the bill directly on the agenda of the senate, bypassing referral to the southern-dominated Judiciary Committee. On March 9 consideration of the bill on the Senate floor and the inevitable Senate filibuster would begin. On March 2, however, the Supreme Court, in an expedited decision, refused to review the *Simkins* case and allowed the Fourth Circuit Court of Appeal discussion on the unconstitutionality of the Hill-Burton separate but equal provision to stand. No one missed the implications for the Civil Rights Bill's Title VI prohibition of the use of federal funds to support racial segregation. As reported in the *New York Times*:

> The high court's announcement was made while the whole issue that was partly involved in the lower court decision was pending in the Administration's equal rights bill on which the Senate had not yet begun debate. Hence the effect of the Supreme Court's refusal to review that decision was to validate as mandatory under the constitution, a hotly disputed section of this legislation in advance of congressional action. . . .
>
> The usual procedure of the Supreme Court is to await the enactment of a legislative draft into law before passing on its constitutionality. In this instance it was known to all concerned—including the Court, which also read the newspapers—that Senate opponents of this particular section (Title VI of the equal rights bill) were preparing a last ditch effort to legislate the exemptions which were outlawed in the lower court decision which it allowed to stand. This being so and in view of the additional fact that the Supreme Court can indefinitely postpone announcing when it will review a lower court decision, it must be concluded that the Court was fully aware that its timing in this case would cut the ground away from the effort in the Senate to maintain in Title VI the exemptions authorized in the Hill Burton Act. . . . In sum, the Court departed from the usual by ruling, not that a statute passed by Congress was unconstitutional, but that a proposal about to be taken up would be if legislated. (Krock 1964, 32)

To a clipping of the *Times* article sent to Cone's administrator, Harold Bettis, the hospital's lawyer attached a note reading, "Harold, this helps explain why we got such prompt 'service' from the Supreme Court" (Roth 1964).

While in the filibuster southern senators tried to portray Title VI as a sinister federal executive power grab, it could now be defended as little more than an obvious rehashing of what the courts had already determined was the law of the land. This outcome would have no doubt pleased President Kennedy, who had approved the intervention of the

Justice Department on behalf of the appellants in the *Simkins* case two years earlier. Fresh in their minds, the *Simkins* case and Greensboro's hospitals were repeatedly invoked by the Senate supporters of the bill in the debate. Finally, the longest debate in Senate history ended, and the bill was signed in the East Room of the White House on July 2, 1964, with most of the civil rights and congressional leaders present. Seven months earlier John Kennedy had lain in state in the same room. Johnson spoke briefly. "Its purpose is not to punish. Its purpose is not to divide, but to end divisions—divisions which have lasted too long. Its purpose is national, not regional. Its purpose is to promote a more abiding commitment to freedom, a more constant pursuit of justice, and a deeper respect for human dignity. We will achieve these goals because most Americans are law-abiding citizens and want to do what is right" (qtd. inWhalen and Whalen 1985, 227–28). Passing the Civil Rights Act had not been easy, and its implementation would prove even harder. More battles would follow. Senator Barry Goldwater (R, AZ), Johnson's opponent in the November presidential election, had opposed the bill, echoing the rhetoric of the Mississippi Sovereignty Commission's Coordinating Committee for Fundamental American Freedom. He argued that the bill will "require the creation of a federal police force of mammoth proportions . . . and an 'informer' psychology, [which] are the hallmarks of the police state and the landmarks of the destruction of a free society" (qtd. in Whalen and Whalen 1985, 213).

Many of Johnson's staff had been aghast that Johnson would take the risk of trying to push through the Civil Rights Bill in an election year while seemingly more important legislation, with much broader public support, such as Medicare and aid to public schools, languished. Many outside Johnson's inner circle just assumed that he had to prove his civil rights credentials to party liberals in order to block a bid to replace him at the Democratic Convention (see, for example, Dallek 1998, 113–15). Joseph Califano Jr., who served as special assistant to Johnson, upon reflection later believed it was all part of "Johnson's plan." "No one understood Johnson's plan. The Civil Rights Act was passed in 1964 BEFORE the enactment of all the domestic programs the following year. No one anticipated the massive flow of federal funding that would begin in 1965. If the civil rights bill had been pushed AFTER all of that subsequent legislation, it would have never passed."[8] Indeed Title VI didn't raise anywhere near the red flags it would have if its enactment had been attempted after all this subsequent federal funding had begun.

Swirling around the enactment of the Civil Rights Act in 1964 were other events more clearly related to the hospital civil rights concerns. On May 15, 1964, Johnson signed the extension of the Hill-Burton Act, with the offending clause permitting the use of funds for the construction of separate but equal facilities deleted. Invited to the signing ceremony, W. Montague Cobb finally had an event worth celebrating. Cobb also participated in another event on July 27, 1964, at least as satisfying. The secretary of HEW and the Johnson administration hosted a conference for top hospital officials related to their responsibilities in complying with Title VI of the 1964 Civil Rights Act, ending discrimination and segregation. Unlike the earlier Imhotep conferences, the top brass of the mainstream associations attended. Secretary Anthony Celebrezze in his remarks thanked the group for coming to discuss ways to eliminate racial discrimination in hospitals: "This is a job that must be done, a job that we in the Government cannot do alone and a job for which I hope you will let us have your help. . . . You are engaged in an important task and I wish you well" (qtd. in Cobb 1964a, 446).

At a January 28, 1965, conference under the auspices of the United States Civil Rights Commission attended by four hundred leaders of all kinds of organizations receiving federal funds, Vice President Hubert Humphrey noted in his keynote address that the law was on the books, and "enforce it we will but we will walk the last mile to assure voluntary compliance" (qtd. in "National Conference on Title VI" 1965). Yet it was increasingly clear both that voluntary compliance would be insufficient to do the job, and that the government had nothing as an alternative.

The picture one gets from reviewing issues of *Hospitals*, the trade journal of the American Hospital Association, during 1964, the year of so many civil rights breakthroughs, was not encouraging. It portrays an insulated world almost oblivious to the civil rights battles surrounding them and determined to keep it that way. The journal's coverage of the Hill-Burton Act extension makes no mention of the elimination of the separate but equal provision, nor do its articles about the need to further strengthen the process of review of physicians for medical privileges in hospitals make any mention of the problem of racial exclusion being challenged in the courts. The only article related to these issues was one appearing in the November 1964 issue that describes the unwelcome intrusion of the Civil Rights Act into hospital operations. The author, the administrator of Methodist Hospital in Gary, Indiana, complained:

> The law creates a fundamental problem for patient care in general hospitals. . . . To legislate that physicians and hospital staffs must ignore emotions in patients arising from any cause is to amend the historical right of medicine to make the patient's wellbeing its most important concern. . . . When patients have predetermined convictions on racial matters, efforts to force changes in them at the time of illness can be detrimental to their medical care. Because the rendering of medical care is a hospital's responsibility, this must be its primary consideration. Difficulties will arise in the implementation of the Civil Rights Act. It is unfortunate that sick people will be asked to face these problems. (E. Johnson 1964, 53–54)

As guidance to the nation's hospitals, this seems more a call to circle the wagons than an enthusiastic endorsement of the intent of Title VI of the Civil Rights Act.

The NAACP Legal Defense Fund would, of course, continue to pursue individual cases of discrimination into the federal courts just as it had done in with *Simkins v. Moses Cone*. In a *Medical World News* article following the Supreme Court's decision not to review the appellate court decision, Legal Defense Fund director Jack Greenberg noted, "We wait to see whether the medical profession will voluntarily follow the law or whether a long hard process of litigation, such as we have had with schools will be necessary." The article noted that many Washington observers "feel that the effect will be gradual, not sudden. Hospital desegregation like school desegregation will have to be fought out case by case" (*Medical World News* 1963, 56). Following the tortuous process school desegregation had followed (and would continue to follow) was not a promising prospect.

Medicare and Title VI

Yet the momentum of the civil rights movement and Civil Rights Act helped propel Johnson's reelection in November 1964, unblocking a flood of legislation. Despite the loss of the "solid South," he beat Barry Goldwater by the largest majority in history. The election also produced a two-to-one Democratic majority in the House and a thirty-two-seat majority in the Senate. It was, among other victories, a victory for the civil rights movement's collaboration with Johnson and an electoral endorsement of the 1964 Civil Rights Act. Almost an afterthought to the civil rights agenda, health care benefits for the elderly now became the easiest gift to provide. Medicare (Title XVIII of the Social Security Act), which had been previously blocked, along with a state-based financing of care for the medically indigent, Medicaid (Title XIX), passed with seeming ease.[9]

Cobb and other medical activists in the NMA had campaigned hard for the health insurance package. This strained their relationship with the AMA even more than their picketing of the AMA's convention in Atlantic City and its Chicago headquarters in 1963. In spite of the spreading culture of protest, picketing was an awkward and uncomfortable thing even for these activist physicians to do, self-conscious about their status in the larger social order. Atlantic City had an ordinance prohibiting placing anything on the boardwalk, and the demonstrators wanted to place their signs on sandwich boards on the boardwalk. "We have these signs and physicians can't carry signs," the organizer explained to the chief of police. "Yeah, you're right, physicians can't carry signs," the police chief answered (qtd. in Smith 1999, 116–17). The protesters were allowed to march around the signs on the boardwalk in their dark suits and ties. The protest focused on the AMA's refusal to require nondiscrimination as a condition for local medical society membership, and a similar protest would follow, the picketing of AMA headquarters in Chicago.

Following the Chicago protest a tense meeting was held in the boardroom of the AMA. The AMA had its own ax to grind. Why had the NMA supported the Medicare legislation when all other doctors in the country supported the AMA's position, the AMA president asked. The NMA was alone among national organizations of physicians in this respect, he argued. Dr. Cobb, present at the meeting as the NMA president elect, observed that "there was no relationship between majority opinion and the truth. Columbus was a unique minority in 1492 in his concept that the world was round" (qtd. in "Third Meeting of the AMA-NMA" 1964).

Dr. Cobb, in return for his organization's support of the Medicare bill, would join President Johnson on *Air Force One* on the trip to sign the Medicare and Medicaid Act at President Harry Truman's library in Independence, Missouri, on July 30, 1965. He was again "a unique minority," the only physician invited to attend. (Truman, still seething from the AMA's campaign against his national health insurance bill, might have blocked the entrance to an AMA representative anyway.) No representatives of the American Hospital Association, Blue Cross, or the commercial health insurance industry were invited to attend either.

The implications of Title VI for Medicare, however, were carefully avoided in the Johnson administration's presentation of the legislation and in the congressional debate (Feder 1977, 12). Senator Harry Byrd (D, VA), chairman of the Senate Finance Committee, in the process of considering the legislation received the following cryptic reply from Secretary Celebrezze to his request for clarification: "I am advised (by the Department's legal staff) that the new hospital insurance program will be subject to the requirements of Title VI" (Celebrezze 1965). While everybody "understood" this, it was in no one's interest to explore exactly what that might mean. What legislation says is one thing; how it is implemented beyond just bland paper assurances is quite another. Indeed, most, perhaps except for the civil rights activists, just assumed it would work just the way school desegregation had worked, with the "all deliberate speed" of the *Brown* decision, and that, at least in the short run, things wouldn't change much. That ambiguity, silence, indeed even secrecy, about Title VI persisted throughout the passage and implementation of the Medicare program.

Those now faced with the complex task of implementing the Medicare program in a mere eleven months would have been happy not to have the issue posed by Title VI. For those in the Social Security Administration who had been attempting to think through the planning of such a program's implementation for more than a decade it was an unanticipated and unwelcomed headache.

The Johnson administration had tried to focus on voluntary compliance. As a few courageous hospitals in the south learned, this didn't work. White flight followed desegregation, punishing compliance and rewarding hospitals that flouted the new law. It became clear that Title VI could not be enforced for hospitals that had already received Hill-Burton funds through federal pleas for voluntary compliance. In the face of hospital intransigence, HEW had few options.

Yet the issue wasn't going to go away. A week after the passage of Medicare, the Voting Rights Act was passed, the culmination of protests that had begun in Selma, Alabama. With the civil rights movement at high tide, neither public officials nor hospitals could expect to be left to their own devices. Either as a way of defusing criticism or building pressure for more effective enforcement, HEW officials privately encouraged civil rights groups to submit complaints. Over the summer and fall of 1965, the Medical Committee for Human Rights (MCHR, a group organized to provide a medical presence at civil rights demonstrations in the South), the NAACP Legal Defense Fund, and the NMA submitted a total of more than three hundred Hill-Burton Title VI complaints. These groups also provided intelligence that would be put to use in developing an enforcement offensive and began a strained partnership that increasingly blurred the boundaries between the civil rights activists and the federal officials responsible for enforcing Title VI.

Three weeks after Medicare and Medicaid were signed into law on July 30, 1965, John Gardner became secretary of HEW. The Voting Rights Act became law on August 6, a triumphant ending to the violent beatings of civil rights marchers by police in Selma and the completion of their march to Montgomery, Alabama. The Voting Rights Act, however, was upstaged three days later by the beginning of the Watts, Los Angeles, riots on August 11.

Johnson had gone from emotional triumph to despair in less than two weeks, and something had to be fixed. As a result, civil rights enforcement responsibilities were decentralized in a directive by Johnson on September 24, 1965, and Vice President Humphrey was removed from any role in the administration's civil rights efforts. Attorney General Katzenbach, a veteran of the school desegregation battles, would serve to coordinate these efforts. In an attempt to avoid criticism from civil rights groups and in a seemingly cruel extra twist of the knife, Johnson demanded that Humphrey present these recommendations as his own, which Johnson was only endorsing to the press (Califano 1991, 64–67). It was a painful, humiliating meeting for Humphrey. No doubt thinking about this specific meeting, he would later describe his meetings with Johnson as an "almost hypnotic experience, I came out of those sessions covered with blood, sweat, tears, spit and sperm" (Califano 2015). Gardner would now have to make sense out of this in the implementation of the Medicare program. There are two possible interpretations of the intent of this directive. First, it would bury the Title

VI civil rights enforcement function within lower levels of the federal executive bureaucracy, giving wide latitude to those directly responsible for overseeing the funding of specific programs and insulating them from much oversight. This was precisely the result the Mississippi Sovereignty Commission's Coordinating Committee on Fundamental American Freedom had feared. Second, it would insulate the president and cabinet officials from any direct responsibility for enforcement, and should any feeble, under-resourced lower-level efforts become a political liability, top officials could protest their innocence, make midcourse corrections, and punish the perpetrators. Johnson probably wanted it both ways, but during the fall of 1965, increasing evidence supported the second interpretation and the civil rights activists' worse fears.

The critical first test of Title VI enforcement's backbone involved a standoff between HEW's Office of Education and Chicago's Board of Education. The Elementary and Secondary Education Act of 1965 passed in April was the centerpiece of Johnson's War on Poverty and influenced by many of Secretary Gardner's ideas. It provided unprecedented billions in aid to schools serving low-income students. The explicit intent was that it would reduce the educational disadvantage of low-income students in schools serving predominantly low-income children. The implicit hope was that it would also help lure southern school districts into compliance with federal pressures to desegregate. Chicago was slated to receive $32 million under the new program (more than $244 million in 2014 dollars). In August, the Coordinating Council of Community Organizations (CCCO), a group representing diverse organizations involved in civil rights activism in Chicago, filed a Title VI complaint with the Office of Education against the Chicago schools, concerning the award.

The CCCO included the local chapter of the NAACP, the Chicago Urban League, and a variety of neighborhood organizations. The focus of their frustration was on the board and superintendent of the Chicago public school system. Residential segregation, selective boundary drawing, and white flight resulted in separate and unequal treatment of black and white children. Just as with the city's hospitals, de facto segregation produced conditions similar to the Jim Crow ones in the South. A protracted lawsuit brought by participants in the CCCO ended in an out-of-court settlement in 1963.[10] The settlement required a report and recommendations from an independent review panel. That panel, headed by Philip Hauser, a demographer and professor of sociology at the University of Chicago, issued its report in March 1964 (Anderson and Pickering 1986, 134). It found that 84 percent of black students were in black schools (schools with at least 90 percent black enrollment) and that 85 percent of white students were in white schools. The degree of segregation was almost as extreme as found earlier in the city's hospitals by the Committee to End Discrimination in Chicago's Medical Facilities. The report also documented the inferiority of the black schools (overcrowding, dilapidated physical facilities, teachers lacking education and experience, and so on). In essence, the public schools in Chicago were as racially separate and unequal as in the Jim Crow South. The report came to similar conclusions as one produced internally for the school board by Robert Havighurst (Havighurst 1964). Faced with the resistance of white communities to any altering of the racial composition of their schools and the resulting resistance of the superintendent and board, none of the recommendations in either report was acted on. The CCCO organized school boycotts and demonstrations to protest the lack of progress, to force a change in leadership, or, at least, to focus national attention on Chicago's school problem.

That national attention came soon. On July 4, 1965, the CCCO, using the information supplied in the Hauser and Havighurst reports, filed their Title VI complaint to HEW's Office of Education documenting the unwillingness of the superintendent and school board to deal with the de facto segregation in its schools. The complaint noted that "the ways and means of perpetuating segregation in Chicago may become the handbook for southern communities seeking to evade the 1954 Supreme Court ruling. We are confident that federal intervention in this matter, through the withholding of funds will help underline the high fiscal costs, as well as immeasurable social costs, of segregation to Chicago and the rest of the nation" (qtd. in Anderson and Pickering 1986, 160). A joint press conference held with the director of CCCO and Martin Luther King on July 7, 1965, and demonstrations in Chicago later in the month added to the pressure. On July 27 and 28, Congressman Adam Clayton Powell held hearings on the de facto segregation in Chicago's schools. A riot on the West Side of Chicago had followed the more destructive one in Watts in August.

The CCCO complaint had arrived amid considerable confusion in HEW about whether Title VI could be applied to de facto segregation or whether it would be more narrowly interpreted to apply only to segregation prescribed by law. That is, could it be applied to the invisible color lines in the North, so well reflected in the segregated hospital care of Chicago and its even more segregated public schools, or did it only apply to the visible color lines of the South? Was the struggle to end racial segregation a national one, or was it simply, as southern critics would argue, one involving a struggle to impose a national will on a region?

US Commissioner of Education Francis Keppel wasn't sure of the answer, but he initiated an investigation. The CCCO in his view had unquestionably submitted a most detailed complaint. Those that read the document were "deeply impressed by the thoroughness and seriousness of the charges" (qtd. in Anderson and Pickering 1986, 178). Keppel and his staff were also irritated by the lack of responsiveness in getting information from the Chicago school system and by the apparent assumption on their part that the funds and their plans for their use were a fait accompli. As a consequence, Keppel sent a letter on September 30, 1995, to the Illinois superintendent of instruction, Ray Page, that the Chicago school system was in "probable noncompliance" with Title VI of the Civil Rights Act. The CCCO complaint "must be satisfactorily resolved before any new commitments are made of funds under federal assistance programs administered by the Office of Education, either directly or through your office" (qtd. in Anderson and Pickering 1986, 179). The $32 million in new funds for the Chicago public schools was put on hold.

The Chicago civil rights leaders were jubilant. For one, the deferral "was another demonstration that the civil rights movement in the city has been telling the truth." Another said he "felt wonderful. I hope that this is the first step toward building a school system that will make every Chicagoan proud" (qtd. in Anderson and Pickering 1986, 180). The federal government, they felt, had vindicated their long-standing claims.

Benjamin Willis, Chicago's school superintendent, was enraged. At a press conference he denounced the federal fund deferral as "illegal, despotic, and alarming" (qtd. in Anderson and Pickering 1986, 179). Congressman Roman Pucinski (D, IL), a supporter of Willis, who chaired the House subcommittee that controlled education legislation, warned that "Congress won't appropriate another nickel for education programs" if federal officials continue such "arbitrary and dictatorial acts" (qtd. in Anderson and Pickering 1986, 176). All of Chicago's and Illinois's congressional delegation backed Willis, including Everett

Dirksen, Senate minority leader who had been instrumental in assuring the passage in the Civil Rights Bill but had assumed that Title VI applied only to de jure segregation in the South.

The response of Johnson was swift. Meeting Mayor Daly several days later at the signing of the new Immigration Act at the Statue of Liberty in New York's harbor on October 3, 1965, Johnson promised immediate action for his political ally (Califano 1981, 220; Anderson and Pickering 1986). The symbolism surrounding this meeting overflows in irony. The Statue of Liberty, erected ten years before the *Plessy* decision, legalizing segregation, had welcomed only white Europeans to its "Golden Door." Up until the 1965 Immigration Act, the United States had denied African and Asian immigration and had given preference to northern Europeans. At the height of the civil rights struggle and after the passage of the Civil Rights Act of 1964, the federal government's own law on immigration was an embarrassment. The importance of this act, signed as a modest bit of overdue housecleaning, was buried in the flood of other Johnson administration legislation. Yet its long-term effects have perhaps been the most profound.[11]

That evening after the signing, Johnson summoned John Gardner, Francis Keppel, Wilbur Cohen, Joseph Califano, Douglass Cater, Johnson's special assistant on educational matters, and Attorney General Nicholas Katzenbach to the White House (Berkowitz 1995, 248–49). He blasted Keppel for not informing Daly, instructed his aide, Joseph Califano, to contact Daly and let him know the money would be forthcoming, and told Cohen to fly to Chicago and work out a secret accommodation. The only individuals who knew anything about the program and the Chicago situation, Secretary Gardner and Commissioner Keppel, were cut out of the negotiating process. Cohen's negotiated deal, releasing the $32 million, essentially turned over the investigation of the CCCO's complaint to the Chicago School Board, the purported defendant in the complaint (Anderson and Pickering 1986, 181). Congressman Pucinski claimed victory, "abject surrender by Keppel—a great victory for local government, a great victory for Chicago. Mayor Daly has done the people of the nation a great service by standing firm against intolerable federal intervention" (qtd. in Anderson and Pickering 1986, 181).

All the local civil rights activists could do was to express their dismay:

We are shocked at this shameless display of naked political power exhibited by Mayor Daly, in intervening at the highest level—not to put Chicago into compliance with the Civil Rights Act, but to demand federal funds regardless of how they are used. Mayor Daly ostensibly supported the Civil Rights Act, all Democratic congressmen from Illinois and Senator Douglas voted for it. Yet they are the first to squeal like stuck pigs when the bill is enforced in the North, while they applaud enforcement in the South. (qtd. in Anderson and Pickering 1986, 181)

It essentially ended any attempt to use Title VI compliance to control the flow of federal educational funding in the North and, for the most part, put it on hold in all areas of the country for the rest of the Johnson administration. Southern school districts and politicians exploited it, blocking desegregation and driving a wedge between the civil rights community and the Johnson administration. An amendment to the Elementary and Secondary Education Act was passed to require uniform enforcement, uniting southern school districts and larger northern urban ones to help undercut aggressive enforcement of Title VI.

Ruby Martin served as deputy to the assistant secretary for civil rights for both Quigley and Libassi and briefly under Cohen as director of the Office for Civil Rights. She was bewildered by Johnson's decision in the Chicago case and dismissed it as probably just a plain case of political interference on the part of Mayor Daly:

> There are some people who suspect that Lady Bird's Beautification Program was at stake, and that Mayor Daly controls eleven votes in Congress, and that he threatened to pull all of them back to Chicago or off the floor when Lady Bird's Beautification Bill came up. I really don't know. Let me say that that was a tremendous setback for us generally because the South seized upon it as we knew they would, and made a political football of it. There are some of us who feel that we would not have had the political problems that we had, had not the Chicago incident taken place. . . . It was an extremely well documented complaint that we had from Chicago. And I know the White House was asked something, either was it all right, or "here are the facts, and we're going to this. Do you have objections?" I think there were just some failures on both sides to follow through.

It would be an awfully good thing to write a book about if anybody could get all the facts. (Martin 1974, 17–18).

Joseph Califano, one observer of the Oval Office confrontation over the Chicago school debacle, laid all the blame on Keppel and his failure to follow the law and use good sense (Califano 1991, 72–74). The problem appears to have been, however, a more complex and nuanced one, as Attorney General Katzenbach, another attendee at the meeting with Johnson, later recalled:

> HEW came into it with a somewhat newer experience and I think a somewhat more heavy-handed way, with school funds, and with less experienced personnel. And we were throughout it trying to get them to adopt the sort of enforcement posture that *we* had of saying, "We're not going to insist on this in schools until we've investigated it all, until we've discussed with you, until we've shown you what the case is, and then you either comply or if you don't, we're going to go to court." . . . HEW didn't really have the same court procedures and to some extent, went somewhat faster with somewhat more difficulties. This happened in some places in the South, but there we really had more experience than they had and when we could find out about it, could bring them into line and show them a little bit more how to do it. . . . They got into this in Chicago and simply didn't follow procedure. And I think that's what irritated the President; it certainly irritated me. This should have been discussed in great detail with all the school people and with Mayor Daley, and it simply had not been. And it was simply done much too quickly with much too little preparation. You'll get that reaction, whether it's Chicago or deep in the Black Belt. (Katzenbach 1968, 19–20)

HEW's problem was, of course, different than the attorney general's problem in bringing school districts into compliance with the *Brown* "all deliberate speed" mandate. The money had to be distributed in an accountable, timely manner. HEW had neither the staff nor the time to realistically adhere to the Justice Department's protocols. The damage, whoever's fault, had been done, and it cast a shadow over the prospects of any effective Title VI enforcement with the Medicare program. During the fall of 1965, the handling of Title VI Hill-Burton complaints appeared to be producing the same inaction as the Chicago complaint about the dispersal of the Elementary and Secondary Education Act funding. The assistant secretary for HEW, James Quigley, was responsible for Title VI compliance but had to rely on existing staff. It was not clear what constituted compliance and, more importantly, how it could be enforced. There was no staff to do the enforcement. The funding for that staff and other resources needed was controlled by Congress. Some of the same Senators on the committee controlling HEW appropriations were the same ones who filibustered against the Civil Rights Bill in the first place. It seemed fruitless to try to get the necessary funding from Congress. Despite all the hysterical warnings of groups such as the Coordinating Committee for Fundamental American Freedom, Title VI was a paper tiger. The "federal police force of mammoth proportions" that Goldwater had warned about a year earlier did not exist. Under Title VI, HEW could levy no fines, could require no periodic reporting, and had no subpoena powers. Individuals could file complaints, but a complaint-driven enforcement system shifts the burden of proof onto the victims, who might well fear retaliation, just as the black physicians in Chicago who had chosen not to bring their concerns to the court-appointed commission responsible for arbitrating problems of racial discrimination in the granting of hospital privileges.

Not surprisingly and in keeping with the attorney general's approach, the Johnson administration focused on encouraging voluntary compliance in the first year after the passage of the Civil Rights Act. At a January 28, 1965, conference under the auspices of the US Commission on Civil Rights attended by leaders of more than four hundred organizations receiving federal funds, HEW secretary Celebrezze pleaded, "We appreciated, particularly, the good faith of all those who have demonstrated an earnest desire to reason with us and work with us in righting these old wrongs. . . . Let no one see, however, in our exercise of reason an absence of resolve to obtain the absolute justice that the law—and our own principles require" ("National Conference on Title VI" 1965, 163). It was not at all clear in terms of hospitals receiving Hill-Burton funds how that "absolute justice" was going to be obtained. A few courageous hospitals, such as Providence Hospital in Mobile, Alabama, had responded to the call for voluntary compliance and desegregated their accommodations (Smith 2009, 37–42). White flight to the hospitals that remained segregated shrunk its census and threatened its financial survival. In the existing local environment those that complied with the new federal law were punished and those that flouted it rewarded. Voluntary compliance wasn't going to work.

The failure of Congress to provide resources for Title VI enforcement had, however, the ironic and unanticipated consequence of shifting control of enforcement into the hands of the civil rights activists. HEW officials, off the record, pleaded with civil rights groups to bring them well-documented complaints and increasingly relied on them for guidance and volunteer staffing. The NAACP Legal Defense Fund, the National Medical Association, and the Medical Committee for Human Rights (MCHR) all began doing volunteer inspections of hospitals in the summer of 1965. These groups and particularly the MCHR provided intelligence about the challenges any compliance process would face and created the rough protocols that would later guide federal inspections. Most of the complaints that had been turned over to HEW for action were from the South. On September 9, 1965, an internal memo from the MCHR secretary to its president indicated the degree of collaboration that was emerging. "I now understand that HEW has need for complaints of racial discrimination from 10 or 20 Northern and Western hospitals. They need them quickly to enable them to get the effect of sudden impact on voluntary compliance on a nation-wide basis since they do not have enough personnel to visit and supervise 9,000 hospitals. The agency confidentially requests that MCHR release the information about complaints to the press since this helps get other institutions in line and the government is much more restricted than a private group in what they can say to newspapers" (Holman 1965). On September 29 another memo from the president to the MCHR secretary instructs her, "Please compile a list of Northern physicians who went South and give it to me immediately. The NAACP Legal Defense and Education Fund has been requested by HEW to seek out physicians who may be willing to go south and make hospital investigations at the expense of HEW" (Parham 1965).

Yet, other than acknowledging receipt of complaints and the other intelligence these groups had supplied, nothing seemed to be happening from the HEW side of this concealed partnership. By December 1965 both MCHR and Legal Defense Fund interactions with HEW had started to get much testier. Alvin Poussaint, MD, southern field director of the MCHR, summarized its concerns in a December 8, 1965, letter to Congressmen Philip Burton, Charles Mathias, Adam Clayton Powell, and Robert Kastenmeier and Senators Jacob Javits and Ted Kennedy:

> During the summer we filed approximately ten complaints of segregation and discrimination in the South to Mr. Quigley's Office. Only one of these was investigated. On a recent trip to Washington DC, I met with some HEW officials who admitted they were not following up complaints adequately. However, they complained that HEW had not been given additional staff to enforce compliance under Title VI. They also state that they had no full time investigators. It appears that enforcement of Title VI has been left to already overburdened staff of regional HEW offices. . . . We hope you will use your influence to aid HEW in obtaining proper resources to adequately enforce Title VI and bring better health services to the Negro, the south and all Americans. (Poussaint 1965)

On December 7, 1965, as a part of a recognition of the growing impasse, Dr. John Holloman, as both president of the NMA and chairman of the MCHR, requested an appointment with Secretary Gardner. Holloman wanted to explore areas where MCHR and its volunteers could enhance "the investigative role of the Department of Health Education and Welfare. Also, organizationally we are giving much attention to action programs embodied in the Medicare Act which we desire to discuss with you" (Holloman 1965a).

The day of the scheduled meeting with Secretary Gardner, not surprisingly, coincided with the submission of a report to the secretary from the Legal Defense Fund, "Report on the Implementation of Title VI of the Civil Rights Act of 1964 in Regard to Hospital Discrimination: Recommendations for 1966." The report noted that while the passage of Title VI should have ended the need for legal remedies, Legal Defense Fund (LFD) lawyers faced "the disheartening task of filing suits against virtually every health facility in the South in order to gain equal treatment for Negro citizens." It further noted:

> The LDF combined with MCHR and NMA have filed more than 300 complaints that have been characterized by Assistant Secretary of HEW James Quigley as "legitimate in that the hospitals in question were totally or partially segregated." The report notes that

"to date, the Department had found only 35 of these in compliance with Title VI. No action has been taken with respect to the remainder despite the fact that many of these facilities have been investigated and reinvestigated by the Department and have refused and are refusing to end discrimination. . . . The Department in no case has sought to cut off federal funds to these hospitals although many are in open defiance of Title VI. When asked to explain why funds had not been cut off, the reply was that the Title VI cut off procedure was too cumbersome to employ. The Department (privately) takes the view that it will be subjected to political pressure if it attempts to move against the hospital. There is no specific appropriation for Title VI enforcement and the personnel who enforce are often borrowed from other programs. A large staff in Washington and in the Regional Offices committed to civil rights is necessary. It is critical that the Department make a firm policy decision that no funds under the Medicare program will be paid to hospitals which are not in compliance with Title VI. To pay these funds to southern hospitals and then attempt to negotiate their compliance with Title VI would throw away a superb opportunity to end racial discrimination in southern hospitals. (NAACP Legal Defense Fund 1965)

For whatever reason (Gardner explained that the appointment had not been confirmed), the secretary failed to keep his appointment with Holloman's group. This precipitated an impromptu press conference, summarizing the LDFs report and noting that the new Medicare program offered "a golden opportunity to wipe out discrimination in Southern hospitals" (Wire Service 1965).

Holloman then fired off a telegram to Secretary Gardner. "We note that you have met freely with conservative elements of the health professions. We wonder if your failure to meet with us had racial implications and may be symptomatic of the reluctance of your department to come to grips with the discriminatory practices in health care. . . . The relative impotence of the Department of Health, Education and Welfare in Title VI enforcement thus far give us grave concern as to the nature of future nondiscriminatory planning and implementation of the forthcoming Medicare program" (Holloman 1965b).

The secretary sent his own telegram back to Holloman indicating that he was unaware of any confirmed appointment: "You may be assured that I welcome your continued suggestions concerning more effective implementation of Title VI of the Civil Rights Act and your cooperation with the department toward that end" (Gardner 1965b). Indeed, it appears that HEW had already begun working off the same script as the activists. Two days earlier, on December 14, 1965, Gardner distributed a memo to every component of HEW, outlining the staffing plan that would be used to enforce compliance with Title VI:

> This is too important to be treated as anything less than the highest of priorities in our total program. The attached plan will work if we set our minds to making it work. . . . The key is adequate staffing. We must assign as large a part of our staff resources to this activity as required to assure effective administration of the Act. It probably will be necessary for the head of some constituent agencies to obtain a specially qualified staff assistant and some supplemental specially qualified staff; however, to the extent possible we should train and utilize our regular staff. From time to time it will be necessary to borrow employees from one operating agency or program to help another. Your full cooperation will be required to make the Department's performance an outstanding one. . . . It will not be possible to consider budget amendments and supplementals; they would not provide the resources soon enough. If, however, the diversion of staff from other activities were to create unmet workload which you consider sufficiently serious to warrant budget action at this time, such request should be submitted for consideration, but only if the problem is significant, the consequence serious, and the need well documented and well-justified. (Gardner 1965a)

Stripped of bureaucratic language, the memo says that HEW is now a civil rights organization, and, as a result, all its employees are civil rights compliance officers. (Gardner was in fact borrowing the idea from Attorney General Katzenbach. After the enactment of the Voting Rights Act on August 6, 1965, Katzenbach immediately drafted federal employees residing in problematic southern states to monitor its enforcement without bothering to transfer budgets or even pay much attention to the wishes of the transferees.[12] Katzenbach was also, as a result of Johnson's civil rights reorganization at the end of September of 1965, responsible for coordinating federal civil rights enforcement.

Gardner must have certainly understood that the attorney general wasn't going to raise objections to an approach to assure adequate staffing for enforcement of Title VI in the implementation of Medicare that he was already using, albeit on a smaller scale, to assure adequate staffing for enforcement of the Voting Rights Act. Indeed, Gardner in his memo is committing all of HEW's existing budget and staff necessary to achieve its civil rights goals. HEW wouldn't waste time trying to get a supplemental appropriation from Congress for additional staff that wouldn't be forthcoming. The memo weaves in the organizational justification offered in President Johnson's September memo, the passionate impatience of the grassroots civil rights activists, and Gardner's own long-advocated vision of individual and national renewal. Its major target, unmentioned, is the new Medicare program just six months away from becoming operational. In effect, it was a call for a volunteer crusade. Gardner was launching perhaps the riskiest domestic policy initiative in the nation's history. It tied together the fate of Johnson's two signature pieces of legislation—the Civil Rights Act and Medicare. It strapped them onto the same raft in treacherous rapids. Johnson, despite political instincts that counseled the caution of a carefully calculated chess game, perhaps not even aware of how it had happened, found himself trapped on the raft as well. There was no turning back, and the raft hurtled over a waterfall with no bottom in sight.

4

"Children's Crusade"

Secretary Gardner and His Memo

Gardner's December 14, 1965, memo must have reached many desks in the HEW bureaucracy with people shaking their heads and muttering, "Is this guy really serious? He can't possibly mean what I think he means!" Even today, it's hard to understand all of what Gardner was really thinking. Federal executive branch departments and their leaders have always been harder to figure than other parts of government. They leave behind less of a paper trail than presidents, legislatures, and courts. The agencies and their civil servants operate in the shadows outside of the public spotlight, implementing presidential directives, legislation, and court orders. Yet in many cases what they do has more impact on what happens. In no case has this perhaps ever been truer than in the implementation of Title VI in the Medicare program. This chapter tries to solve the mystery of how they were able to accomplish so much with so little and in so little time.

Gardner meant all that was implied in his memo. He was, of course, in part responding to the pressure of the civil rights groups and the furious urgency of a president convinced of both the broader cause and the shrinking window of opportunity (Califano 2015b). In the wake of the Watts Riots, Johnson knew that time was of the essence. White support for Civil Rights was shrinking and black impatience exploding. Yet Gardner wasn't just responding to these pressures. He believed in an individual and national transformation shaped by the vision of the civil rights movement and that Medicare's implementation offered the best opportunity to begin to realize it.

In this regard, Medicare's implementation had the advantage of being a back-burner issue as far as the president, the legislature, the press, and the general public were concerned. Its passage had been sandwiched between the Elementary and Secondary Education Act and then the Voting Rights Act and Watts Riots. School desegregation, voting rights, urban riots, and the escalating Vietnam War seemed far more volatile and pressing concerns. The implementation of the Medicare program just seemed a technical matter, best left to the experts. Johnson's domestic policy aide Joseph Califano recalled the White House devoting very little attention to Medicare's implementation (Califano 2015b). It was almost as if it were on autopilot. Part of the lack of attention reflected the deference given by the White House and the general public to hospitals and medicine. That deference, just as it helped make black physician and dentist leaders of the local civil rights movements, now helped insulate Medicare's implementation process from top-level executive and legislative interference. The Johnson White House just assumed that the professional service ethic of hospitals and physicians was compatible with the administration's civil rights goals and would deliver the desired results without producing any explosive political problems (Califano 2015b). The reorganization of federal civil rights enforcement efforts at the end of September 1965 helped reinforce such an approach, giving Gardner more of a free hand in staffing enforcement. This set the stage for a remarkable transformation of the nation's hospitals. That deference and delegation, however, as many critics have subsequently noted, was far less successful in designing a payment system that would control costs and a quality assurance system that would really protect Medicare beneficiaries (see, for example, Reinhardt 2015).

Gardner, assuming the position of secretary of HEW on August 18, 1965, just several weeks after the enactment of Medicare, was an interesting choice by Johnson. HEW had a reputation for being a difficult agency to run. According to Califano, Gardner was chosen in the hope that he would help attract the people needed to engineer the transformation envisioned in Johnson's Great Society programs (Califano 2015b). Those programs would flow through supportive legislative committees on the Hill and into HEW to administer. Gardner, described by some as a radical in pinstripes, baffled Washington. He seemed to live on a kinder planet lacking Washington's political and bureaucratic cynicism. Meeting at the White House shortly before Gardner took the job of secretary, a Johnson staff member shook his head afterward in disbelief: "He thinks like a saint." "No," Johnson replied, "he thinks like a good Republican. They're harder to find than saints. And besides, one is all you need" (qtd. in Moyers 2003, xiv).

Gardner, frustrated novelist turned academic psychologist and then private foundation president, took the job after a relatively contemplative one at the Carnegie Foundation overseeing a staff of thirty-six.

As HEW secretary, he oversaw 106,000 employees spread across competing bureaucratic empires. Gardner had caught the interest of Johnson because of his work exploring ways to improve education for low-income children. He had no experience working with hospitals, which may have been just as well; he would have been much more reluctant to commit the resources to the Title VI hospital compliance campaign. He brought with him the optimistic, some would say naïve, tenets espoused in his books, such as *Excellence: Can We Be Equal and Excellent Too?* and *Self-Renewal: The Individual and the Innovative Society*. In none of his writings and speeches are the words "segregation," "discrimination," or "race" ever used. Yet these were the central problems he wrestled with during his tenure as secretary. He preferred to focus on universal hopes, not what divided people. "What we have before us are some breathtaking opportunities disguised as insoluble problems," he observed in taking on the job of HEW secretary (Moyers 2003, xv).

Gardner was no mystical visionary. He recognized that his first task as secretary was to recast its story in a more favorable light. "Our goal is to proctor human fulfillment within a framework of values and laws. We deal with the obstacles to human fulfillment whether poverty, or ignorance, or sickness, or trouble with the police. We are the department of people," he explained (Gardner 2003, 14). That didn't eliminate HEW's image problems, but those that worked there liked the sound of it. Reflecting on his time as secretary, "In Washington," Gardner wrote, "the person who rushes to put out every minor blaze is 'someone who gets things done.' If he pauses to think about next week's fire, he's an 'impractical visionary.' If he strikes a pose as he pours water on last week's dead ashes, he's a statesman" (Gardner 2003, 18). He let eight to ten key subordinates cultivate their own access to White House staff rather than controlling access himself. The advantage was that it allowed him to learn more about all the intricacies of White House staff relationships and shifts in priorities. The risk was that you lost control. Gardner was willing to take that risk, even after the Title VI disaster with Mayor Daly and the Chicago public schools. That mistake was not repeated with Title VI approvals for hospitals to get Medicare funds. Marvin Watson, an old Texas political confidant and friend of Johnson, served as his the key political watchdog on Title VI matters involving hospitals. Gardner and Johnson had mutual respect and trust. Their friendship outlived Gardner's eventual resignation after he concluded that Johnson could no longer lead the country and should not stand for reelection. It was a conclusion that Johnson would come to himself several months later. This relationship and Gardner's deferential, non-confrontational style assured him a free hand in managing departmental initiatives. His views on leadership as a way of fostering individuals to achieve their full potential may have helped generate the renaissance of creative problem solving among those engaged in the Medicare civil rights enforcement effort. They all ended up being unorthodox, inventive risk takers. Only one thing, as far as Gardner was concerned, was of critical importance:

> I had to put in place the first enforcement of the civil rights legislation. The more I studied it, the more apparent it became that we had to be utterly consistent. What we were doing was forcing a fairly deep change in a culture by coercion, by legislation. We were saying, "there's a piece of your culture that you've got to root out." This was serious business. Even someone who believed as deeply as I did in the cause had to recognize that this was tough stuff. The least you could do was be absolutely clear and consistent as to what you wanted. There remained inconsistencies within the administration itself. If I got the slightest wind of it, I'd jump in my car, go and see the person involved and say, "You know, it's very tough to administer this, we've just got to hold the line." It worked. (Gardner 2003, 24)

Gardner made it clear to his subordinates, reflecting the basic message he was getting from Johnson and the White House, that there could be no fudging because of the time or political pressure. He tried to make sure other departments in the executive branch, the Justice Department, and others, also held firm. A united front was critical or the whole offensive would collapse. Keeping the lines of communication open between him and Attorney General Katzenbach, now responsible for coordinating all federal civil rights enforcement activities, was a major concern. The case of the Daly and Chicago schools disaster was still fresh.

Gardner's major adversaries in terms of Medicare civil rights enforcement were the southern senators and congressmen. He would meet regularly with Senator Richard Russell (D, GA), a leader of the southern coalition opposing desegregation who had filibustered against the Civil Rights Act. Russell was also the powerful chairman of the Senate appropriations subcommittee that HEW's budget depended on. Sessions with him were always courteous and civil. At an early meeting, Gardner reported that Russell told him, "Well you understand, Mr. Secretary that I'm just dead against what you're doing. I think it's bad for my state, bad for the South and it isn't good public policy." Gardner responded, "Well I understand that, I understand what's going on. I realize that we are, in fact, coercing many of your people to follow a path which they've not traditionally followed. But I have to remind you that I'm doing it to enforce the law that came out of this institution. The Senate and the House passed this law, I'm enforcing it, and, as long as I'm Secretary, I will continue to enforce it" (Gardner 2003, 21). Gardner later reflected about his dealing with Congress that "below the surface there is a deep suspicion of the executive branch, a fear that the bureaucrats will out-maneuver them, cover up, evade and get their way" (Gardner 2003, 20). Such a fear among southern legislators was well founded in the case of Gardner.

Gardner's Team

In mid-December 1965 Gardner appointed Peter Libassi to work closely with him as special assistant for civil rights. Libassi's recruitment was prompted by the Chicago embarrassment and intended to assure control over the HEW's decentralized Title VI enforcement efforts in the secretary's office.[1] Libassi had worked from 1956 to 1962 as regional director of the New York State Commission against Discrimination. In that capacity he was responsible for overseeing investigations and hearings related to discrimination in employment, housing, and public accommodations in the upstate New York region. That experience resulted in his recruitment as assistant director and then deputy staff director of the United States Commission on Civil Rights in Washington, DC, in 1962. At the time, there was no comparable federal operation accountable for addressing discrimination. Just as the Social Security program in the 1930s had borrowed from Roosevelt's efforts to put a similar program in place as governor of New York, the Commission on Civil Rights perhaps hoped to borrow again from New York's experience with Libassi's help. Libassi had been responsible at the commission for investigating problems of discrimination in federal agencies. He would now join Ruby Martin, a former colleague at the commission who had been involved in developing its reports on school desegregation, in the secretary's office. The US Commission on Civil Rights had been a critic of HEW's efforts in addressing discrimination, and putting its critics to work on the inside made sense to Gardner.

Libassi, however, was a latecomer to the tightly knit team making preparations for Medicare's implementation. His intrusion with a new agenda could hardly have been welcomed. Two talented career bureaucrats, Wilbur Cohen and Robert Ball, had responsibility for turning the Medicare Care Act into an operational program enrolling and serving more than twenty million seniors, providing payment for services from about eight thousand hospitals, 250,000 physicians, and a complex array of other service providers. The clock was ticking, and they now had less than six months to complete the job.

Wilbur Cohen, deputy secretary at HEW, had begun his government career in 1934 in the New Deal and had well earned the title "Mr. Social Security," also the title of a biography about his life (Berkowitz 1995). He knew the intricacies of its laws and regulations and was a consummate negotiator. As Theodore Marmor, who served as an assistant to Cohen during the period of Medicare's implementation, observed, "Wilbur Cohen's office was like Grand Central Station. Nothing bureaucratic about it—no layers and a wide range of players."[2] It included freewheeling exchanges and discussion with industry leaders such as Walter McNerney, president of the national Blue Cross Association. White House aide to Johnson Joseph Califano observed, in a forward to Cohen's biography, that he knew "it's important—and enough—to move the ball down the field; it's not necessary—or possible—to score a touchdown on every possession" (qtd. in Berkowitz 1995, xi). Johnson understood this as well and had relied on Cohen to patch things up with Daly and the Chicago public school Title VI confrontation. Gardner later appreciated these same qualities in Cohen, recalling a time when a confrontation over a regulation loomed with a key legislator. Cohen advised simply withdrawing the regulation, reworking a few words in consultation with the legislator. This produced the needed result (Gardner 2003, 21). The two, however, had different priorities. When Gardner left HEW, along with Libassi, to join the Urban Coalition, Cohen succeeded him. For Secretary Cohen, the effective operation of Medicare, Medicaid, and other HEW programs was the most important priority (United States Commission on Civil Rights 1970, 10–11). For Gardner, it was all about achieving the cultural transformation represented in the Civil Rights Act.

Robert Ball, commissioner of social security, formally reported to Cohen. Both had worked together in the Social Security Administration for many years, and Ball was given a free hand in handling all the details of implementing the Medicare program. He would later reflect, "There was almost complete delegation of authority and responsibility to the Social Security Administration from higher levels. I don't think I can exaggerate the degree of this, the thought from above was: we are not going to try to, in any way, interfere with the agency's sole responsibility to put this in effect" (Gluck and Reno 2001, 10–11). Ball had been the chief administrator of the Social Security Administration since 1953. Son of a Methodist minister, he obtained a master's degree in labor economics in 1936. He worked for several years in the labor movement before joining the Social Security Administration in 1939, doing the pedestrian fieldwork of helping employers set up accounts for their employees. It was not a popular program then. Both employers and employees viewed it as a tax, and, given this lack of public support, Congress had little interest in expanding it. His rapid rise in the Social Security Administration reflected his contributions in transforming it into an expanded and popular program with broad bipartisan support. Given Ball's knowledge of the details of the Social Security programs, his deferential nonpartisan approach, long-tenured and loyal team of experts, and large field staff, no one challenged that delegation.

Libassi's responsibility in the secretary's office was to coordinate civil rights enforcement across all the different agencies and programs administered by HEW. The largest challenge he faced was the enforcement of Title VI in the implementation of Medicare. It was there, unnoticed by other key actors in the implementation of Medicare or at least unchallenged by them, that a profound shift in Title VI's enforcement policy took place. The assumption apparently up until then of legislators and the White House was that Title VI would work just the way it had worked for public schools, adopting the "all deliberate speed" approach that had been used to "implement" the *Brown* decision. Title VI enforcement using such an approach would have been no big deal.

Hospitals would just submit a plan just as school districts had. A few token gestures would be required, but real desegregation could be delayed indefinitely.

Three experienced, forceful individuals on Libassi's staff reflected the growing consensus of the civil rights movement. They argued for the abandonment of the "all deliberate speed" approach with hospitals seeking participation in the Medicare program. Ruby Martin had preceded Libassi from the US Commission on Civil Rights to the secretary's office and was still furious about the Chicago school cave-in. Sherry Arnstein had worked with James Quigley, Libassi's predecessor in the secretary's office, in dealing with hospital Title VI Hill-Burton complaints and had been directly involved in forcing the desegregation of medical school hospitals. (She had been sent to the University of Mississippi medical center to certify their compliance with Title VI soon after the passage of the Civil Rights Act to assure the flow of NIH funding in response to Executive Director Marston's request.) Arnstein was the most knowledgeable and perhaps staunchest advocate of the new approach to desegregation on Libassi's new team. Derrick Bell was recruited by Libassi in January 1966 to serve as legal counsel for Libassi's new team. He had served in the Justice Department's Office of Civil Rights in the late 1950s before being pressured out because of his refusal to give up his NAACP membership. Bell had then joined the staff of the NAACP Legal Defense Fund under the direction of Thurgood Marshall before returning to the secretary's civil rights office. He would later become Harvard Law School's first black tenured professor and the widely acknowledged founder of critical race theory.[3] All three argued that there should be no "all deliberate speed" pass for hospitals wishing Medicare funds. No money should go to any facility where race played any role in treatment of patients, employees, or medical staffs. NAACP and National Medical Association leaders had also pressed Gardner for such an approach. Libassi, the newest recruit to the Title VI struggles with hospitals, respected and accepted their advice.[4] According to Libassi, no one up the chain of command (although some may not have been aware of the major shift in approach until it was too late) questioned it either. "No one said no. They were afraid of the risks it involved but unwilling object."[5] Libassi's team had, in effect, rolled the dice and it was now up to everyone else to deal with the consequences. Not surprisingly, according to Marmor, "there was real tension between the old order Social Security group responsible for implementing Medicare and Libassi. Title VI (at least in the way it was now being used) had not been a part of their game plan."[6]

The Social Security Administration had no experience in enforcing Title VI requirements. It managed its own programs, and program payments went directly to beneficiaries. This would prove a distinct advantage in administering the Medicare program. The Social Security Administration, however, did have a well-established administrative infrastructure for dealing with appeals from prospective beneficiaries who had been denied eligibility for benefits. It involved an appeal to an administrative law judge, transcripts of the resulting hearing, and a final administrative decision. A prospective beneficiary, not satisfied with that decision, could then, and only then, pursue the address of their grievance in the courts. In effect, with the Medicare program, hospitals became prospective beneficiaries as well. Rather than lose Medicare payments and pursue the delayed and dubious prospects for a successful appeal, it just made more sense, for all but a stubborn few, just to comply with the requirements.

The actual task of certifying Title VI compliance for hospitals wanting to participate in the Medicare Program fell to the Public Health Service. The Public Health Service administered the hospital Hill-Burton program and was already deeply immersed in dealing with the complaints that civil rights activists had brought against hospitals. That experience, combined with the need to avoid duplication, made the Public Health Service the logical place to locate the hospital compliance effort.[7] Like the Social Security Administration, the Public Health Service operated programs across the nation and had a long history of working with local and state health departments. William H. Stewart, MD, who had previously worked closely with Wilbur Cohen in crafting the Medicare legislation, was appointed surgeon general in September 1965. He served as head of the Public Health Service, one of the uniform services, also holding the anachronistic title of vice admiral. Stewart appointed a career officer in the Public Health Service, Leo Gehrig, MD, as deputy surgeon general, assigning him responsibility for the oversight of Medicare Title VI compliance for hospitals. Appointed under Kennedy, Gehrig had previously served as the first medical officer of the Peace Corps. The actual work of certifying Title VI compliance was assigned to the Office of Equal Health Opportunity (OEHO), established in February 1966. Its director, a social worker from New Hampshire and a career civil servant, Robert Nash, had assisted in drafting the HEW's Title VI guidelines. OEHO had a staff of five. A faceless bureaucrat, Nash would remain so. Robert Ball, social security commissioner and director of Medicare's implementation, confessed later that he had never even met the man.[8]

The prospects were not encouraging. It would be easy to conclude that the Title VI Medicare enforcement initiative would never be heard from again. What, after all, could a handful of inexperienced staff in an office buried well down the chain of command possibly do to transform eight thousand fiercely autonomous and politically savvy local hospitals in four months? Yet the entire civil rights movement had been propelled by idealistic high school, college, and young adult volunteers beginning with no organization at all. Few of its leaders were over thirty. It had been a children's crusade. What if this fledgling organization tapped into the same pool of youthful idealism and launched its own "children's crusade"?

The Short Happy Life of the Office of Equal Health Opportunity

The Office of Equal Health Opportunity (OEHO) began its short, happy, heroic life in the Public Health Service in February 1966. Its mission was to enforce Title VI compliance for any hospital wishing to receive Medicare payments. Hospitals, according to policy established by the civil rights group in the secretary's office, could not just offer bland assurances of their good intentions, as had been tolerated with public schools systems in the South and northern cities such as Chicago. As of July 1, 1966, they had to be fully, genuinely racially integrated. OEHO's director, Robert Nash, had participated in the interagency taskforce that pulled together the regulations on what that meant. In creating guidelines for hospitals the task force used all it had learned from civil rights group complaints against hospitals. The guidelines, as Gardner had insisted, were concrete, comprehensive, clear, and consistent. They stated:

> Hospitals in compliance with the Act are characterized by absence of separation, discrimination or any other distinction on basis of race, color or national origins in any activity carried on in, by or for the institution affecting the care and treatment of patients. Specifically, the above would include (but not be limited to) the following characteristics:

1. The hospital provides inpatient and outpatient care on a non-discriminatory basis; all patients are admitted and receive care without regard to race, color or national origin. Declaration of an open admission policy may not be sufficient to effectuate compliance in some instances, particularly where the hospital has previous served only or primarily patients of one race. Where there is a significant variation between the racial composition of patients and the population service area, the hospital has a responsibility to determine the reason and to take corrective action if they are due to discriminatory practices.

2. All patients are being assigned to all rooms, wards, floors, sections, and buildings without regard to race, color or national origin. In communities with non-white population, this results in bi-racial occupancy of multiple rooms, wards and use of single bed rooms on a nondiscriminatory basis. Patients are not asked if they are willing or desire to share a room with a person of another race. Transfer of patients is not used as a device to evade compliance with the Act.

3. Employees, medical staff and volunteers of the hospital are assigned to patient services without regard to the race, color or national origin of either the patient or employees. Courtesy titles (Mr., Miss, Dr.) whenever used are being used throughout the hospital including patient care areas and news releases announcing admissions, births, deaths, etc.

4. The granting of permanent or temporary staff privileges is carried out in a non-discriminatory manner. Staff privileges are not denied professionally qualified personnel on the basis of race, color or national origin or on the basis of non-membership in an organization which discriminates on the basis of race, color or national origin. Removal of staff privileges and other disciplinary actions shall not be based on race, color or national origin.

5. Non-discriminatory practices of the institution includes all aspects of training programs and require recruiting and selection of trainees at both predominantly white and Negro schools. The same recruiting procedures are used at all such institutions. Third parties are not permitted to select trainees on a basis which, if done directly by the hospital, would be

violative of the Civil Rights Act. These requirements apply to interns (medical, dental, OT, PT, dietician), residents and training programs such as graduate nurse, practical nurse, medical technology, X-ray technology, etc.

6. All services rendered by the institution, its employees or vendors to patients or others are provided without regard to race, color or national origin. This would include:
   a. Administrative services (admission, medical records, fiscal, etc.).
   b. Medical and dental care for inpatients and outpatients (all specialties—clinical, diagnostic and other pathology services).
   c. Paramedical care and ancillary and supporting services (food, pharmacy, social services, laundry, toilet facilities, waiting rooms, entrances, exits, snack bars, gift shops, visiting hours, doctor's lounges). Patients and visitors are using all cafeteria facilities without regard to race, color or national origin; no dining facilities are used only by non-whites by "custom" or "preference."
   d. Ambulance services.
7. Employees and medical staff have been notified in writing of the hospital's policy for compliance with Title VI of the Civil Rights Act.
8. Hospitals which have recently changed from discriminatory practices have taken steps to notify those who have previously been excluded from hospital services (e.g. letters to Negro physicians or physician organizations and Civil Rights leaders, notices to newspapers, posting of signs in hospitals, etc.).
9. Hospitals which have had dual facilities to affect racial separation have either converted one of them to a different purpose or have taken steps to change the traffic flow so that they are actually used bi-racially. ("Title VI and Hospitals" 1966)

Who, however, would assure that hospitals certified to receive Medicare payments consistently adhered to these guidelines? More than four thousand hospitals were clearly out of compliance, many resistant to becoming compliant. Gardner had sent out the request for temporary transfers to OEHO, but who, if any, would volunteer for such a thankless, hazardous assignment, and how could they possibly produce such a fundamental transformation in such a short time?

Just in the way the mysterious voice in the film classic *Field of Dreams* said, "Build it and they will come," they came. An odd collection of passionate idealists emerged from the maze of HEW bureaus and departments and trickled onto OEHO's "field." That field was hidden in the Social Security office complex outside Baltimore. OEHO could accept as many temporary transfers from other parts of HEW as it could use. No one was "assigned" this duty. Just as the Freedom Riders, lunch counter demonstrators, and marchers in Selma had, they just showed up. Hearing about it from other activists or reading Gardner's memo, they just went to their supervisors and requested the transfer. Most of these volunteers were already involved as civil rights activists and jumped at the opportunity.

The federal government, like private organizations, temporarily transfers employees all the time. In most cases a few people are transferred to help deal with an unanticipated temporary technical problem. This was different. Nothing of the size of this temporary transfer had ever happened at HEW before nor has happened since. Altogether about one thousand civil servants participated in this temporary transfer. Roughly half came from the Social Security Administration and the other half from the Public Health Service. Few had any experience that was even faintly relevant to the task that they were now expected to perform. The recruits included bench scientists from NIH, veterinarians, pharmacists, managers of Social Security field offices, venereal disease investigators, even a "medical officer from the Indian Health Service complete with an Eskimo secretary."[9] Added to this mixture were sixty medical students who volunteered for it as a summer job. In its conception, the Title VI inspection team for a hospital was supposed to include a Public Health Service medical officer in uniform, a local social security office staff person, and a representative from the newly created regional civil rights enforcement group, but the actual inspections that were carried out, given the time constraints, rarely fit such an orderly, full staffing pattern. The teams and individuals doing the inspections were uniform only by their passion for the civil rights cause. It was a children's crusade, and any objective prediction would give them less chance of succeeding than the original one in the Middle Ages.

Robert Nash was the right field commander for this passionate volunteer bureaucratic army. He told one of his recruits, "If I don't want to take on a hospital, I'll refer it to General Counsel for advice. Three months later they'll get back to me with a reason why I shouldn't do anything. If I want to take on a hospital, I'll just use my own lawyer and do it."[10] The logistics of managing this army were bewildering. Peter Libassi, whose office was responsible for coordinating all Title VI enforcement efforts, was located in Washington, DC, in the HEW north building on the Mall below the capitol. Most of the offices handling the OEHO Medicare campaign were distributed across four separate buildings in the Social Security complex in Baltimore. The field operations, however, were spread out over eight regional offices across the country.

Frank Weil, one the more experienced early recruits, had a perverse gift for handling these logistics. He had served as national secretary for the American Veterans Committee (AVC). The AVC had been formed after World War II and, unlike other veterans groups, specifically focused on desegregation and in addressing progressive causes. Medgar Evers had written a letter of acceptance to join the AVC board the night before he was murdered. Weil had worked to arrange for his burial in Arlington so at least he could laid to rest in an integrated cemetery. He worked on civil rights efforts related to integrating bars and restaurants around military bases in Mississippi in the summer of 1964. "I got shot at but they missed, although Hertz was somewhat miffed when I turned in a car with bullet holes."[11] His experiences during the brief life of OEHO were magical ones for Weil, for whom nothing was impossible, and even the most audacious approaches to solving problems got results.

> I showed up in Baltimore at Social Security, where we were going to set up operations. That same morning an emissary from Commissioner Ball's office came and asked, "What do you need?" I said, "I need about six lawyers, and I've found that your switchboard doesn't know we're here and I've had difficulty getting calls." "Well, as to the lawyers," he said (he looked at his watch and it was now about 11:00 AM), "do you mind if they don't report until after lunch?" I said, "No, I don't mind at all, thank you." The next morning there was a phone on my desk that was so direct I didn't have to dial 9.
>
> After about six weeks we needed to decentralize the files, which were all in Baltimore and we needed to get them to the regional

offices where they could be used. The day we needed to do this, there was a civilian pilot's strike, and we couldn't send them by airmail. We were able to get the files to Charlottesville and New York by car but the other regional offices were too far. I got an idea. I didn't consult with any one, I just did it. I told six senior public health officers on my staff to go home and put on their uniforms. We cut military orders for them and sent them up to Andrews Air Force Base in a truck with the files. We cribbed orders similar to those used by the Pentagon and had the surgeon general sign them with his alternate title Vice Admiral. Nobody was going to question the orders of a Vice Admiral, particularly if you couldn't understand the initials after his name! The next day the other six regional offices had their files.[12]

Yet underneath all the official pronouncements about progress in achieving voluntary cooperation, not much had changed. A report by the US Commission on Civil Rights in January 1966, after review of the files on complaints submitted by Civil Rights groups to HEW and a survey of thirty-nine southern and border state hospitals, had concluded that at least two-thirds were substantially out of compliance (United States Commission on Civil Rights 1966). More troubling, the report noted that cases where one hospital in a community had taken steps to integrate, it had lost admissions of white patients as physicians chose to admit them to the hospitals in the community that remained segregated. Not only did this threaten the financial viability of hospitals that chose to comply with the law, but it would increase the resistance of hospitals that had yet to desegregate. In addition, many hospitals in northern cities that had escaped notice since they had all signed the HEW nondiscrimination assurance forms (Form 440) operated as de facto segregated facilities. Few had done much to force changes in their institutional culture. Medical staffs still excluded qualified black physicians and, as in Chicago, informally understood not to admit their black patients to the historically white facilities on the edge of ghettos where the physicians had privileges. In addition, admitting clerks still often placed black patients on the charity wards even when they had private insurance. Most of the hospital guidelines for Title VI were in practice flouted in the North as well as the South. Whether OEHO Title VI compliance effort could do much to change all this in less than four months seemed dubious, and the political backlash that would result from denying access to care to elderly Medicare beneficiaries at the hospitals in many communities would be ferocious. Maybe, to use Califano's football analogy in describing Assistant Secretary Cohen's acumen, they should just punt to move the ball down the field and worry about scoring the touchdown later.

As plans went ahead, everyone assumed that there would have to be a final Johnson decision about whether to proceed. Most former OEHO staff members assumed that Gardner had to have met with Johnson sometime in February to get the final approval. The risk to the Johnson administration and its two signature pieces of legislation, the Civil Rights Act of 1964 and the Medicare and Medicaid Act of 1965, was just too great. They were on a collision course. There is no record of any meetings where this might have been discussed. It is plausible, given the Johnson administration's delegation of both civil rights responsibilities and Medicare's implementation as well as all the other pressing matters the White House was dealing with, that there never was such a meeting and that, rather than a "decision," the Johnson administration had been trapped through all the incremental decisions described here so that any kind of retreat was no longer an option. In effect, this test of wills was the domestic equivalent of the "decision" to pursue a costly war in Vietnam, and the prospects seemed less promising.

On about March 1, 1966, Joseph Califano requested that Peter Libassi meet with him at the White House. "How are things going Pete?" Califano asked. "It's going well, except there are not going to be any hospitals in the South certified for Medicare." Startled, Califano asked, "What do you mean?" "There is no 'all deliberate speed' for hospitals, they have to be fully integrated to receive Medicare payments," Libassi answered. After a long pause, Califano said, "OK, let me get back to you on that."[13] Califano never got back, and plans proceeded. One can imagine that Johnson, in keeping with his stubborn ambition, may well have responded to this wakeup call saying something like "I want the southern hospitals in Medicare, I want them to comply with the civil rights requirements, and I want the Medicare program to begin as planned. Do it." The "decision," or at least the decision not to interfere, had been made. The federal government, no matter what the consequences, had left "all deliberate speed" far behind.[14]

On March 4, 1966, the highest-stakes poker game in health policy history began. Under Surgeon General Stewart's signature, a letter went out to every hospital in the country ("Title VI and Hospitals" 1966).

Dear Hospital Administrator:

Title VI of the Civil Rights Act of 1964 prohibits discrimination on the basis of race, color or national origin in Federally-assisted programs. To be eligible to receive Federal assistance or participate in any federally-assisted program a hospital must be in compliance with Title VI. The Public Health Service has been given the responsibility of ensuring compliance with Title VI in all hospitals receiving funds directly or indirectly from any department or agency of the Federal government. . . . Enclosed is a description of the requirements of the Civil Rights Act as they apply to hospitals. (The Hospital Guidelines.) Also enclosed is an Assurance Form 441 to be signed, indicating your compliance with the conditions of Title VI. This form will need to be signed and returned in order to participate in direct Federal programs such as Health Insurance for the Aged. . . . The questionnaire is in addition to what you may have already provided to a state agency. . . . We will review the questionnaires as they arrive, and if any deficiencies are noted we will let you know so that you can take any necessary action to correct them. . . . Representatives from the Department of Health Education and Welfare Regional office will be visiting hospitals on a routine periodic basis to supplement this information and to be of further assistance in resolving any problems that may arise. . . .

Sincerely yours,
William H. Stewart
Surgeon General

No one—the Medicare implementation planners, the civil rights activists, the Department of Justice, the Public Health Service Team now responsible for hospital Title VI compliance, the die-hard segregationists, the hospital boards, or the hospital administrators—was sure what was going to happen next.

Just three weeks later on March 25, 1966, Martin Luther King Jr., the keynote speaker at the Second National Convention of the Medical Committee for Human Rights in Chicago, noted in his summation, "Of all the forms of inequality, injustice in the health care is the most shocking and inhumane."[15] It was a recruitment pitch for volunteers to join the upcoming battle, and some of the key recruits were in the audience.

"The Two-Day Wonders"

The first challenge was to prepare the diverse group of volunteers joining the crusade. OEHO needed investigators who would follow a standardized protocol, do it quietly, and accomplish the implausible goal without stirring up a hornets' nest.

Given the time constraints, limited familiarity with what the volunteers might face, and even more limited knowledge about how best to prepare them, they launched the compliance offensive on a prayer and a two-day workshop. OEHO conducted the first two workshops at the Center for Disease Control in Atlanta, April 4–5 and April 6–7, 1966. Speakers, guests, program staff, consultants, and the compliance officer trainees packed into the meeting room. It was not the typical two-day conference brought together by government- or hospital-related groups at the CDC to explore ways to tackle a health problem. There were no medical society representatives or hospital administrators, board members, medical chiefs, or industry consultants present. The invitees included representatives from the full array of civil rights groups—the Student Non-violent Coordinating Committee (SNCC), the Southern Christian Leadership Conference (SCLC), the Southern Regional Council, the National Urban League, and the National Association for the Advancement of Colored People (NAACP) (Hess 1991). The consultants who assisted in the development of the training session and would continue to assist with the compliance effort included five members of the Medical Committee for Human Rights (Drs. Alvin Poussaint and Marion Cunningham from Mississippi, Allen Kaplan from Tennessee, Wilmetine Jackson from Georgia, and John Holloman from New York City, then president of the NMA). In addition to Holloman, MD, the NMA consultants who would assist with the investigations included Hubert Eaton, MD, and Charles Watts, MD. Representatives from church groups and labor organizations who had been active in civil rights efforts were also invited to the sessions and to serve as consultants. The rest of the participants were government officials and volunteer trainees.

Not surprisingly, given the attendees, the meeting began with a debate about whose meeting it was (Childers 2014). The civil rights activists argued that the goal was to crack down on all hospitals that discriminated, while the government officials argued that the job was to determine full compliance only for those hospitals that had chosen to participate in the Medicare program and had signed the Title VI assurance form. (As it turned out, since almost all hospitals ended up choosing to participate, the debate was more philosophical than practical in its implications.) In effect, however, it was the civil rights activists' meeting. They would prove to be the final arbiters of Title VI compliance. A common criticism of government regulation is that it too often leads to regulatory capture by the industry being regulated. Hospital Title VI compliance for Medicare, however, had become perhaps a unique instance of regulatory capture, not by the industry being regulated, but by a social movement seeking to transform it.

An additional training session for volunteer transfers was held in Dallas on May 12, 1966. The Atlanta and Dallas regional offices included all the southern and border states that it was assumed would be the most problematic. A final training session was held later in Washington, DC, for the sixty medical student recruits. The crash courses outlined the civil rights law and regulations, the duties field compliance officers were expected to perform, and the procedures to follow in conducting the hospital site visits and in soliciting supplemental information from the local minority community. Some of the volunteers never attended these training sessions and were just thrown into the fray to learn on the job. Most of the trainees had accepted ninety-day or shorter details to OEHO.

At the White House there was now growing realization of what a high-stakes gamble they were now committed to and that it might not pay off. In the South there could be large areas where Medicare beneficiaries, both black and white, would have no access to hospital care. Johnson was now pressuring Gardner for results, and the pressure at all levels became intense. On April 8, Philip Lee, Gardner's assistant, recalled a meeting, the only time he saw Gardner really angry. Bob Ball, Wilbur Cohen, and other senior HEW officials attended the meeting, and Secretary Gardner "let us know in no uncertain terms that he was not satisfied with the progress that had been made up to that time; that he wanted us to devote whatever resources were necessary to assure maximum compliance on the part of hospitals. . . . The Secretary was absolutely firm in his decision that we would not compromise with the requirements, the issue of Civil Rights was too important to compromise" (Lee 1969, 1–2, tape 2).

Trial by Fire

Nothing, however, could have prepared HEW officials or their volunteer recruits for what lay in store for them. Many of the Social Security Administration recruits had an advantage over the others. They were southerners and were familiar with the challenges faced by forcing desegregation in the South. Two to three years earlier a memorandum had been sent out from Commissioner Ball's office that the Social Security Administration would no longer service "contact stations" (places, usually municipal or county facilities, where Social Security staff would meet on a periodic basis with beneficiaries or applicants for benefits who needed assistance) that had segregated drinking fountains or restrooms. About seven hundred contact stations, mostly in the South, had such segregated accommodations. "I was the field manager in Florida and we would visit the Flagler Contact Station and their restrooms and water fountains were labeled "White" and "Colored." We told them we were not going to come any more unless they changed that. The feeling I got was that they wanted to change but didn't want to do it because of public pressure. So that they would say, we don't want to do it but the feds demanded it. And they did change." Of the seven hundred problematic contact stations only three in the end had to be closed, but it was a drawn-out and acrimonious process (Hess 1991).

How was that change in the contact stations possible? A combination of factors helped: (1) the direct action and other pressures applied by local civil rights groups on both local and federal public officials, (2) the pressures of the Kennedy administration to accomplish low-profile civil rights results, and (3) the unique niche occupied by the Social Security Administration at the time. It was held in high regard by the general public and had gained broad bipartisan support in Congress. It fostered a high morale and close identification with its mission among its workforce. It also had successfully dealt with the racial discrimination issue in desegregating its own offices in the South in compliance with Truman's executive order. Those offices had become tiny islands of integration in the Jim Crow South. They were tolerated because the alternative of not having a local Social Security office, from the perspective of the local community and its politicians, was worse. When push came to shove, preserving the color line was never an intractable battle. It depended on what one got in return for eliminating it. Eliminating segregation in return for preserving convenient access to Social

Security services was a price in the end most local community officials were willing to pay, particularly if it could all be blamed on the federal government. Hospitals, however, are much more resistant to federal pressures to change than local governments. It would be, as these Social Security Administration temporary detail volunteers to OEHO knew, a trial by fire, and time was running out.

One of the new recruits who worked in the Baltimore headquarters for the campaign recalled a common problem.

> We'd go to work in the morning in Baltimore and by 9:15 two or more mornings a week there would be a phone call, and one of our investigators had been stuck in jail—the usual charge was driving a stolen car. What they did was, whenever a rental car was late being returned, the rental car company files a stolen car report. When the car is turned in, they file another report saying the car was returned. The local police department keeps active the first reports but does not act on the second. They know you're coming, and they make sure you get one of the "stolen" ones. Sometime he doesn't make it to the hotel. Sometime he does and they just arrest him if he's difficult on the visit to the hospital—if, for example, he asks to see the chart of the patient in the biracial room, who is really one of the physician's maids. If the gracious lunch at the country club doesn't make you less persistent, the next time you get in the car you get jailed. Sometimes the detailed "volunteer investigator" the veterinarian or the dentist from the Public Health Service would panic.[16]

The game of harassment and intimidation of the federal inspectors could sometimes get more threatening. One inspector was shaken by an incident in Tuscaloosa, Alabama, when almost all the lugs were removed from her right front tire during a hospital visit. Only a freak snowstorm that slowed her return drive to the airport prevented a serious accident (Rose 1997). A Social Security Administration detailed investigator born and raised in Selma, Alabama, recalled that in the midst of a polite meeting with the administrator of a small rural hospital in Mississippi, the administrator paused and said, "I called some of the boys in the KKK when you arrived. I didn't know you were going to be such a nice fellow, you better leave while you can."[17] He left in his brand new Oldsmobile speeding as fast as he could. Even those in the

Baltimore headquarters assisting hospitals in getting Title VI certification were not immune from threats. "I was the only person that could sign off. People would call about why their certification had been held up. You'd explain and give them your name in case they had further questions. My name was in the telephone directory so it wasn't hard for any of these callers to find out where I lived. They'd say, "Oh you've been so helpful." I had a five foot cross burned in my front yard. I wasn't there but I heard about it from my neighbors."[18]

In many cases, old habits would trip up the efforts of hospitals to conceal discriminatory practices. In one case, before visiting a small Alabama hospital, an inspector stopped by the local coffee shop.

> While he was sipping his coffee another man came in and took a seat near him. The counterman came up and said, "How are things goin' George?" George said, "Oh, not so good. Some of those civil rights workers are coming to look at the hospital today. But I've got things fixed up so that we will be able to pass inspection. I put some Negroes in over in the white ward and some white patients in with the Negroes. I told some of our colored workers to come down and eat in the cafeteria today."
>
> Our team member, a distinguished looking gentleman with a mustache and a habit of wearing distinctive vests, cleared his throat several times so the hospital administrator looked over toward him. Some 45 minutes later, when our man walked into the hospital administrator's office he was treated—in his own words—to the most "classic double take" he had ever seen. As hospitals came to realize that we would return to look into complaints these instances occurred more and more rarely. (Nash 1966a, 248)

Another investigator recalled a similar double take while meeting with the nun who was the administrator of a Catholic hospital in Nashville.

> She was insistent that her hospital was in compliance and it probably largely was. I sat in the office and she got an in-coming telephone call. It was from the admissions office and she talked about having a black male bed up on or a black female bed up on so and so, and then she realized I was sitting in the room and she was terribly embarrassed by it. Clearly they had segregated wards

and she had done lots to lead me to believe that they didn't. (Plotz 2000)

The Ritual Dance

In most cases however, it was more a ritual dance where both understood what the outcome would be and, whatever the ambivalence, accepted it. The southerners on detail from Social Security were the best partners for such a dance. The hospitals had all signed the assurance form and knew what was at stake.

> If they tell you they will do it, they will do it. These are people that will come to a full stop at a stop sign in the middle of the night. Bill Stewart and Bob Nash were from North Carolina and understood. We are talking about dollars not about morals. The hospital program was implemented quickly. . . . Our message was: Don't do it unless you mean to comply. You won't be able to hide noncompliance and it makes things worse for you. They had asked to participate and indicated their willingness to comply with the civil rights act. It would amount to up to sixty-two percent of the money they would receive, so it was a big incentive. (Childers 2014)

The administrators understood that it was about more than just getting the Medicare dollars. Segregation created all kinds of headaches and inefficiencies for a hospital. One of the inspectors got called by the hospital administrator in Tupelo, Mississippi, pleading to be put to the head of the queue. "The hospital had gone from nothing to a beautiful establishment. He wanted me to come up and inspect it. 'You can talk to the board and I can't,' he said. I didn't pass them. I told them when they got pure of soul I'd come back."[19] Being "pure of soul" was not something that one could find anywhere in the regulations, but the board got the message. Another inspector recalled doing inspections at rural hospitals in the Dallas region.

> Talking with the Administrator and his board or with the Administrator and other employees . . . they would rant and rave about the beds and the governmental intervention and all that. Finally the board would say "we've got to have the money."

Everybody would glumly say "OK." But then later we would be talking with the administrator in private . . . they would say, "I'm so glad you stopped me from having to run two hospitals here." (Hess 1991, 12)

Even Arthur Hess, deputy director of Social Security, got involved in some of this kind of action. "I didn't get into many of the hospitals except some of the big Southern Baptist hospitals. I dropped in one and we went through with the Administrator and Board and they were ranting and raving but as we were leaving, one board member came up to me and quietly said, 'keep the heat on'" (Hess 1991, 12).

Behavior Not Paper, STAT!

The guidelines said that if a hospital wanted Title VI certification to receive Medicare there could be no difference in the actual way blacks and whites were treated by a hospital—STAT (immediately)! No assurances of good intentions, no plans for future racial accommodations would be acceptable. In other words, there could be no informal or self-segregation of blacks and whites in a Title VI–certified hospital. You couldn't just remove the "Colored" and "White" signs from the entrances and bathrooms and let things proceed as they always had as suggested by the Mississippi Sovereignty Commission to the University of Mississippi Medical Center in Jackson. You couldn't just argue that people "preferred" or "felt more comfortable" self-segregating by race. The inspectors would return and insist on physical changes in the space that would give no one such a choice. In one case that meant not just removing the signs on entrances that said "White" and "Colored" but in one case relabeling them "Entrance" and "Exit" and fixing the hardware on them so that you could only enter one and exit the other.[20] At Windsor County Memorial Hospital in North Carolina the problem of self-segregation in the dining areas was resolved by removing all the tables and chairs in the smaller, historically "colored" dining room and locking the door (OEHO 1966). In another hospital inspectors found removing the signs in the emergency room waiting area was not sufficient. The solution prescribed by the inspectors and implemented by the hospital resulted in placing a rope barrier to one of the waiting rooms and a sign reading "OVERFLOW WAITING ROOM, TO BE USED ONLY WHEN THE MAIN WAITING ROOM IS FULL." Integration could not be left to the preference of patients or staff, particularly in communities where there was the potential for retaliation. There could be no "freedom of choice" or "free market decisions" when it came to being a Title VI–compliant facility.

The vast majority of the hospitals chose to comply in order to get the Medicare payments, and it was remarkable how fast and dramatic the changes were. Two telegrams arrived at the same time from the same North Carolina community, one from the all-black hospital and one from the all-white one. "What should we do?" the two telegrams asked. "Merge" was the one-word telegram sent by OEHO in response. On their own and over a short interval, that is what they did.[21] OEHO official Frank Weil got word from civil rights activists in Louisiana that even though most of the individual hospitals were making an effort to comply, the Louisiana Red Cross Blood Bank still segregated the blood provided to Louisiana's hospitals, labeling them "White" and "Colored." "I didn't check to see if we really had the authority to do it, I just sent a telegram to the Director of the Louisiana Hospital Association that, unless this policy was changed, ALL the hospitals in Louisiana would be out of compliance with Title VI."[22] No litigious protest followed. The Louisiana blood supply was integrated overnight. "We were really doing something. We really felt useful," Weil reflected.

The Acid Test

The acid test of Title VI compliance, random room assignment, worried some hospitals, federal officials, and legislators. Racial separation had been a part of the hospital and medical experience of seniors all their lives. What would happen if they woke up after a life-threatening admission sharing a room with a person of the opposite race? As Frank Weil, one of OEHO's policy makers, explained, "We wanted to reform people, we didn't want to kill them."[23] A May 13, 1966, letter to the board chairman of Albemarle Hospital in Elizabeth City, North Carolina, a community bordering on the Atlantic coast and the state of Virginia, from Robert Nash tried to clarify the federal position.

> We realize that many patients have been accustomed for years to discriminating against Negroes—it is just the way they think they are expected to behave. A hospital cannot eliminate discrimination in services and at the same time follow a policy which routinely

accommodates to the customs of discrimination of individual patients. If such a policy is followed, the logical results are separate hospitals, separate floors, separate units and obviously segregated and usually inferior services. A hospital needs to discourage the exercise of these customs in the hospital by following a clear policy of routinely disregarding race in assigning accommodations. I fully realize that a policy of not honoring patient's requests for transfer on racial grounds is one which cannot be completely rigid in its application. It is not our intention, for example, to interfere with the judgment of the patient's physician, nor prevent the exercise of good judgment on the part of the hospital administrator with respect to obviously troublesome cases. What we would like as a general principle, the medical needs of the patient and not his race dictate the accommodation he occupies and that transfer of patients not be used in such a way as to negate the results of the basic room assignment policy. What we must look for and judge is a demonstrated intention and ability to fulfill the spirit of the Federal Act; and while this necessitates positive, and sometime firm action on the part of the hospital, it does not rule out the application of good old common sense. The possibility of a traumatic relationship developing between patients and instances in which a patient's medical condition would be adversely affected by the presence of a patient of a different race in the same room or ward are not prevalent enough to have any appreciable effect upon the end results of a policy otherwise conscientiously applied. We hope that this explanation will be helpful to the Board of Trustees and enable you to overcome this one remaining difficulty. (Nash 1966b)

A copy of the letter was sent to North Carolina senator Sam Ervin. It was also circulated as guidance to all eight OEHO regional coordinators for resolving the problem of patient "reassignment."

In September 1966, after the main battles were over, Senator John Stennis (D, MS), tried to lead a belated southern counter attack against the Medicare Title VI compliance effort. He inserted a provision in the appropriations bill for HEW that would permit hospitals to continue to segregate patients by race if, in the opinion of the patient's physician, his medical condition would be adversely affected by racially integrated accommodations. Some northern senators predictably expressed concern in the debate that it would create a loophole large enough to "drive a Mack truck through" (qtd. in Reynolds 2004, 719). The provision was defeated, but Stennis did get a gracious letter of assurance from Secretary Gardner that this would be the case. OEHO staff was pleased since they had already put together a form for the physician to sign and knew what the consequence would be. Most physicians don't like filling out any more forms than they have to, and they also didn't like being placed in the position of legitimizing racism as a medical condition requiring special treatment. Patients and families requesting such transfers were typically greeted with a reassuring but stern response from their physician that they would be perfectly fine in the room they had been assigned and times were changing. Few if any forms were signed, and a miraculous national cure of the complicating medical condition of racism resulted.

Indeed, overall, it became hard to figure out what the fuss had been about. Even the earlier court-ordered forced desegregation of Atlanta's public hospital, Grady Memorial, passed almost unnoticed despite the fears of its administrator.

> On the night of June 30, 1965, we moved the patients all around. We just came in to rooms and wards and said, "You're being transferred to room so and so." We just pushed the beds around. I was scared to death. I couldn't talk about it. I didn't know what would happen. We didn't make any public announcements about it. Of course, the director of nursing and the chiefs of services were told. I thought we were going to have a terrible time. There were going to be pickets, maybe even a white uprising against the hospital. Not one damn thing happened. The next day, the papers simply announced that integration had taken place, "in perfect order."[24]

No patients at Grady complained. The breakfast trays arrived and the other hospital routines proceeded as if it had always been this way. Underneath the surface calm, however, there were initially a lot of frightened patients. A director of nursing at a retirement community in Connecticut recalled how frightened her grandmother had been. A patient at Grady at the time, she was told that they were going to "move her to the other side." Her new white roommate was just as frightened.[25]

Yet the early days of integration of hospital accommodations broke down color lines well beyond the boundaries of the hospitals. Raleigh-Durham surgeon Dr. Charles Watts recalled one of his black male patients shared a room in the newly integrated hospital with a white patient who also loved baseball. They watched the games together on TV while recovering from their surgery. The two became close friends attending minor league games and family barbeques together after discharge. He also recalled two elderly women who shared a room and became friends. One took care of the other after discharge until her relatives could arrive to help care for her. These enriching interracial friendships would have never happened without the random room assignment requirement.[26]

OEHO's Hidden Army

If there could be debate at the early training sessions of hospital investigators over whose meeting it was, there could be no debate about who actually directed the inspection and Title VI certification process. The local civil rights activists worked closely with the OEHO inspection staffs, and they became a well-coordinated team. It was a complaint-driven process that relied heavily on local leaders of NAACP chapters, local members of the NMA, and black hospital employees. These local volunteer participants guided the inspection process, and their judgments bore the most weight in recommendations sent to Baltimore on Title VI certification for the hospital. They knew best where all the skeletons were buried, and administrators and hospital boards soon learned, as a result, that it was impossible to conceal discrimination and segregation in their facilities from the OEHO investigators.

> We went to a very large hospital in Louisiana which had filled out the little one page form alleging to be fully integrated. I went with an investigator (Bruce Lowe) who still works in the Office for Civil Rights in Dallas. We go to this laboratory. He opened the door of the refrigerator and the blood was labeled "black" and "white." Then we got into the nursery. It was fully integrated. So we felt better and figured the blood could be corrected. And I thought everything is OK so let's go home but Bruce wasn't happy. So that night we went out to visit some of the employees in their homes. We visited a lady who had been looking after the nursery during the day. She said, 'I'm, so glad you came. Do you know what really happened? Mrs. Smith came running down the hall and said Mary, the Feds are coming, get those babies together. As soon as y'all left she came in

and re-separated the babies." We didn't certify the hospital that day! (Hess 1991, 11)

The hospital had to be visited several more times before they gave up attempting these compliance charades and fully integrated the patient floors. In many communities black hospital workers played a critical and risky role in keeping the certification process honest. They could lose their jobs and possibly face other forms of retaliation. The investigators did everything they could to protect the confidentiality of these local informants. Local hospitals knew the inspectors were coming and did everything they could to prevent unsupervised access to their black employees.

> You would go into a town and you would immediately be followed
> by state police or local cops. A lot of the lower-paid employees in
> hospitals were blacks, and you couldn't be seen talking to these
> people or they would be fired the next day. . . . You would make
> arrangements secretly in advance. You'd go into something like the
> local dry goods store. The cops usually wouldn't follow you into the
> store, or, if they did, you'd go into the ladies lingerie department.
> A cop in uniform was usually unwilling to go into ladies' lingerie,
> and you'd go down the stairs and out the back door, and your
> contact would take you to the meeting. There, the local NAACP or
> a church group, would meet with you and with some of the black
> employees of the hospital. They'd go over the floor plans of the
> hospital with you and show you where the black lunchroom was,
> and you'd learn other things, like the doctor who would bring his
> maid to occupy a bed and so forth. You'd then go on the visit and
> the hospital administrator would take you on a tour. You'd go down
> to the basement where you knew the black staff cafeteria was, and
> he'd say, "Well, why don't we go this way?" and you'd say, "No why
> don't we go this way." You'd then walk into the shabby black staff
> lunchroom. . . . We knew we had to be selective about where we
> went if it all was going to get done. We'd call on black physicians
> to help. Dr. John Holloman, who was president of the National
> Medical Association, was hired on a part-time basis and would
> spend a day a week with us making calls to local physicians in the
> South to find out the problem spots. We'd talk to the network of

civil rights organizations. We relied to a large extent on contact with community groups.[27]

In essence, given the time constraints and the lack of familiarity of inspectors with the day-to-day functioning of hospitals, local civil rights activists ran the show. The resolution of their complaints and their approval drove the Title VI certification process. The interviews with black community leaders were a central part of the protocol of inspectors. In the case of Windsor County Memorial Hospital, North Carolina, the inspection in April 1966 included interviews with key black leaders, including those who had submitted Title VI complaints about the hospital. The hospital had previously closed the black entrance and had eliminated room assignment by race. A field interview with the local black undertaker helped shape their recommendation.

> His statement in substance was: "The Changes made at Windsor County Memorial Hospital are 'terrific.' I wouldn't have believed it had I not seen it myself. If anything, the hospital is now 'too integrated' in that the hospital in making random assignment of rooms has placed some mighty unwashed Negroes in rooms with very fine whites. The entrance problem has been solved. The dining rooms are open to all. If the dining rooms are not being used on an integrated basis, I doubt that it's the hospital's fault. Rather, the Negroes on the staff may be holding back to let someone else be the 'trailblazer.' The changes in attitudes and policies of the hospital and the fact that the hospital has implemented the new policies are generally known throughout the local Negro community." . . . Both Mr. G. and I were impressed with the manner of this informant and believe he is forthright and sincere in his statement. (Department of Health, Education and Welfare 1966)

On May 6, 1966, the acting coordinator, OEHO, Region III (Charlottesville, VA), submitted his recommendation with the full report to the acting chief of field operations in Washington. He suggested that Windsor County Memorial Hospital was operating in compliance with Title VI. Its certification as a participating hospital in the Medicare Program followed soon afterward.

The Golden Rule

Hospitals, for the first time, faced a choice. They could choose to comply with Title VI and receive Medicare and Medicaid payments for their patients that would account for more than 50 percent of their revenues, or they could refuse. With rare exceptions, most hospitals in the 1960s faced looming deficits as the cost of the care they provided grew while the ability of their patients to pay for it didn't. As many as half their patients were over sixty-five. Voluntary health insurance for such high users of hospital care was unaffordable for most. Medicare payments to hospitals offered a golden opportunity out of this bind. For most it meant the difference between expanded services and increased profitability or decline, insolvency, and closure. Boards of voluntary hospitals are responsible for protecting the assets entrusted to them. They are self-perpetuating and not accountable to public officials or an electorate. Such governance had previously helped insulate them from pressures to desegregate their medical staffs and accommodations. That same insulation now protected them in taking what, in many communities, would have been the politically suicidal steps in assuring full compliance with Title VI. The "golden rule"—those with the gold ruled—applied. Implausible as it may now seem, the Medicare program was the first major test for the federal government in applying that rule.

When reports of lagging compliance in Texas hospitals got to Marvin Watson's desk at the White House, they got special attention. Watson wanted to head off potential political embarrassment for Johnson that might undermine the whole effort and reflect poorly on his boss. He requested that OEHO follow up with Marshall County Hospital in Lady Byrd Johnson's home county. Dr. Richard Smith, a former Peace Corps volunteer, made the trip as a special envoy of the president. He was greeted at the airport with an unnerving escort of pickup trucks with shotguns. His day-long session with the hospital's authorities had not budged them an inch. "Fine," Smith finally said in exasperation, "but you just tossed away $100 million in Medicare funding" (Tidwell 2000, 28). A week later Smith was called by the hospital's board chairman. "The trustees had just fired the Administrator and wanted to know what they needed to do to desegregate and get the Medicare money." It was a decision arrived at, in one way or another, in almost all hospital board rooms across the country. Those with the gold ruled.

The Final Days

By the beginning of May, Johnson's phone began to ring. The message from southern friends about the Title VI hospital desegregation effort was always the same: "They won't Lyndon, you know that. Do you want to be responsible for closing St. Francis Hospital in Biloxi, Mississippi? That's what will happen if you put this thing into effect. They're not going to change their ways overnight. You know that as well as I do. Doctors won't treat the colored, and nurses won't treat them" (qtd. in Miller 1980, 412).

On May 6, 1966, Libassi sent a memo to Special Assistants to the President Joseph Califano and Douglass Cater as well as Attorney General Nicholas Katzenbach (Libassi 1966). In twelve southern or border states less than 50 percent of the hospitals had been certified for participation in Medicare. Some of the remainder had not replied to the original inquiries, and the rest had not corrected discriminatory practices. In Georgia only 16 percent had been approved, in Virginia 11 percent, Louisiana and South Carolina 10 percent, and Mississippi only 3 percent. The July 1 deadline loomed, and Califano, presumably at Johnson's direction, scheduled a meeting with all the top officials in HEW and the Justice Department.

A memo from Douglass Cater to the president on May 19, 1966, reflects the growing unease. Cater urges a rethinking of the approach to school desegregation, describing Title VI as a "faulty instrument which Congress added to the Civil Rights Act largely to keep Adam Clayton Powell from adding it to every piece of social legislation that came along" (Cater 1966). The weaknesses Cater ascribes to it in dealing with school desegregation could apply equally to hospitals. Perhaps he and other White House staff had just prematurely written off the use Title VI as a "faulty instrument" in health care as well.

A White House staff memorandum to the president from the director of emergency planning on May 23, 1966, reflects the growing concern and uncertainty over whether the bluff of Title VI enforcement was really going to work with southern hospitals.

> You asked that I review the circumstances as of July 1 when Medicare becomes operative in relation to hospital availability under potential civil rights limitations.
>
> For practical purposes compliance with Title VI by hospitals

will be complete in all States except Alabama, Louisiana, Mississippi and South Carolina. Alabama and Mississippi are probably not to be greatly improved; Louisiana and South Carolina may be.

Options are limited:

1. Civil rights requirements be waived for an additional period of time on the proposition that the health of the people is the first consideration. Such a waiver would obviously encourage resistance.
2. Refuse financial assistance in some more recalcitrant areas as a demonstration that resistance will not be allowed and, for the moment, ignore other non-compliance.
3. Ban all financial assistance to all non-complying institutions. . . .

Secretary Gardner and his staff are doing all that can be expected and may gain additional success before June 30. Governor George Wallace is now trying to get the Southern governors to a meeting and is encouraging hospitals in his own State to refuse compliance. Where there are gubernatorial elections, his conduct poses a real problem. . . .

I recommend that a final course of action not be determined until we are closer to June 30, to give Secretary Gardner's force maximum opportunity to succeed. I do not believe we need fear a "scandal" that might have resulted from nation-wide non-compliance. (Bryant 1966)

Gardner's "force" was pulling out all the stops, but the sheer mechanics of getting so much done in so little time was overwhelming. As one Atlanta regional office employee temporally transferred to the OEHO effort noted later, "as of June 15th in the City of Atlanta we had only 39 beds officially certified for Medicare. It scared the hell out of me" (Hess 1991, 8). The Baltimore OEHO group was now working around the clock. "Everyone worked eighteen to twenty hours a day. We used a hotel room near Social Security just to shower and change clothes."[28] Frank Weil, responsible for the final certification of hospitals for Medicare in Baltimore took up residence. "I moved a cot into my office and put my marriage on hold; fortunately it survived."[29]

Vice President Humphrey called OEHO in Baltimore and asked if there was anything he could do to help, even if it was just checking forms.[30] According to a June 18 memo from White House aide Douglas Cater to President Johnson, Humphrey had made calls to the mayors in Baton Rouge, Greensboro, Knoxville, Houston, Jacksonville, and Dallas asking for their help with the hospitals in their cities, and he was expected to complete calls to the cities in Alabama over the weekend. "He reports that the Mayors have been uniformly appreciative of this effort and are ready to cooperate," Cater noted (Cater 1966).

Lyndon Johnson was now fully engaged as well and using all his magical skills to subject laggard hospitals to the "Johnson Treatment." On June 3, Johnson received the Award of Merit from the National Council of Senior Citizens in the Rose Garden of the White House. Busloads of senior citizens from all over the country arrived at the White House gate to participate in the event. Johnson used the occasion to turn up the heat. "It is fitting that we should come together once more on the eve of a great new era for older Americans. Next month the medical program that you and I labored so long and so hard for will become a cherished reality. . . . I have asked you this morning—you and every one of your local organizations to get in there and help all you can. Alert your hospitals to the requirements of the law, particularly the nondiscrimination requirements of Title VI. Encourage them to meet those requirements" (L. Johnson 1966b, 1). On June 15 at a White House meeting with hospital leaders from across the country Johnson was more direct:

> Never before, except in mobilizing for war, I think, has any government made such extensive preparations for any undertaking as we have made in connection with medical care. . . . Now we know there are going to be problems. One of them arises from compliance with the laws of the land, specifically the Civil Rights Act. In some communities older people may be deprived of medical care because hospitals fail to give equal treatment to all citizens and they have discriminatory practices.
>
> Well, we believe the answer to that problem is a simple one and that Congress has given it in the law itself. We ask every citizen to obey the law.
>
> A majority of hospitals—we think now more than 80%—have already assured us that they will. And I am hopeful that most others—when it is understood and when it is explained—will make an attempt to come into compliance. But we cannot rest easy as

long as any of our older citizens lose their rights because of hospital defiance or because of delay.

Now we are going to hear about those cases. Mr. Rayburn, who served here 50 years, used to say that it is typical of the American people to give more recognition to a donkey that will kick a barn down than a carpenter that will build one.

That applied to all our people. And to those who still stand outside the gates I want to say this: Please comply. If you discriminate against some older citizens in your community, then you make it very difficult for the whole program.

The Federal Government is not going to retreat from its clear responsibility and what the members of Congress have written into the law. And I hope that you will not retreat either.

So you are here today to help us make this reality clear to your communities. Because there is always a last minute hope that we can "fudge it" a little bit and we can prolong it and "it won't be necessary." Now that is one problem and it is a serious problem for the 20 percent group, as you can see. (L. Johnson 1966a, 1–2)

Peter Libassi, who had provided White House aide Douglass Cater with a lawyerly brief explanation of Title VI to be included in the president's remarks to the group, was thrilled to hear his words come from the mouth of the president, who at the lectern seemed to tower over his hospital audience. With the usual pride of authorship, Libassi thought his words were brilliant. "Then Johnson stops in the middle of his presentation, he takes off his glasses and points them at the audience with a stern expression, '*I want you to know, we ain't gonna lock the barn door after the hoss has been stolen. We're gonna desegregate the hospitals!*' No one in that audience remembered my words and no one forgot Johnsons!" (Berney 2015).[31]

Johnson may have upstaged Libassi with this rhetorical flourish, but it set in concrete the principle created in Libassi's office that had driven HEWs entire Medicare Title VI certification effort: there would be no "all deliberate speed" for hospitals, and nothing short of full desegregation and an end to discriminatory treatment would be acceptable. Johnson's performance, however, was mostly preaching to the choir. Few of the hospital representatives attending the session hailed from the southern states that included most of the 20 percent of problem hospitals. Dr. Jean Cowsert, medical director of Providence Hospital in Mobile, Alabama, was that city's lone representative, a city in which all four of its hospitals had yet to be certified. She would soon launch a lonely battle against a far more impenetrable barrier to compliance, the nation's medical profession.

The medical profession had been left out of the Title VI compliance battle imposed on hospitals. A provision in Title VI of the Civil Rights Act had excluded its application to federal "contracts of insurance." The intent had been to allay the fears of some southern senators that Title VI would be applied to federal insurance on bank deposits and might be used to block bank mortgages to housing that was racially discriminatory. (The passage of the Fair Housing Act of 1968 seemingly rendered the concession to allay this fear irrelevant.) HEW's general counsel, however, applied this insurance exemption to Part B of the Medicare program that paid physicians. It was a debatable decision but a practical one since it would have been hard to figure out how it could be applied to private medical practice, particularly given the opposition of organized medicine to the "government run" Medicare program. An effort to delay implementation of Part B in order to exert greater control over the program, including provisions for Title VI compliance, lacked support in Congress. Johnson was able to get an extension in the enrollment period through Congress for the physician payment part of the act, but both still commenced on July 1, 1966.

After Medicare's passage, however, organized medicine remained an obstacle. The AMA had opposed the act, and many feared that it would refuse to cooperate in its implementation. The Ohio Medical Association, representing more ten thousand physicians, had already voted on a resolution to boycott the program. At the AMA national meeting, attended by some twenty-five thousand physicians in June 1965, its House of Delegates directed its officers to meet with the president about the program's implementation. Rumor of a nationwide boycott was in the wind, and some of the association's officers mulled such a step as they traveled to the July 29 meeting at the White House (Woods 2006, 572). AFL-CIO president George Meany, who had learned of the upcoming meeting, called Johnson, fearing either a physician boycott or concessions that would destroy Medicare. "George, have you ever fed chickens?" Johnson asked. "No," Meany answered. "Well," Johnson said, "chickens are real dumb. They eat and eat and never stop. Why, they start shitting at the same time they're eating and before you know it, they're knee deep in their own shit. Well the AMA's the same. They've been eating and eating and now they're knee deep in their own shit and everybody knows it. They won't be able to stop anything" (qtd. in Dallek 1998, 210).

Indeed the AMA delegation arrived ill prepared to deal with a vintage Johnson "treatment." The president launched into passionate praise of American medicine, about how fond he had been of his own family doctor, and how the doctor had cared for his mother and father during long illnesses. How he was sure his respect for doctors was shared by all Americans. Medicine was a noble profession, the noblest of all. In the midst of this flattery, Johnson changed course. Would the AMA help arrange for physician volunteers to serve for short periods in Vietnam to help the civilian population gain a modicum of health? "Your country needs your help. Your President needs your help." In unison the delegation responded that they would be glad to help. "Get the press in here," Johnson shouted to his press secretary Bill Moyers. To the journalists the president announced the commitment of the AMA to send volunteer physicians to Vietnam and praised their patriotism. One of the reporters, perhaps prepped beforehand, asked if the AMA intended to boycott Medicare. "These men are going to get doctors to go to Vietnam where they might be killed. Medicare is the law of the land. Of course they'll support the law of the land. Tell him," Johnson responded in mock indignation, gesturing to the head of the AMA delegation. Flustered, the physician responded, "We are, after all, law abiding citizens and we have every intention of obeying the new law" (qtd. in Califano 1991, 50–51). Several weeks later, the AMA announced its willingness to assist in the implementation of the Medicare program. Not only did the session shift the center of gravity in medicine toward participation in the Medicare program, but it resulted in more than five hundred physician volunteers providing care in Vietnam before the end of the Johnson administration. The irony is the support resulting from a distraction in a well-designed persuasion outlived all the political support Johnson gained from passing Medicare in the first place.

Yet "the chickens," borrowing from President Johnson's AMA story, were now coming home to roost. Medicare's new beneficiaries still lacked access to Title VI–certified hospitals in wide swaths of the South. At the beginning of June 1966, Medicare reported that more than 80 percent of the nation's hospital beds were in compliance. That statistic glossed over the southern resistance and made the accomplishments look better, since the larger hospitals tended to fall into compliance sooner (for example, teaching hospitals and larger hospitals in metropolitan areas). "It was a shrewd public relations position because the hospitals that were still out were a bit timid. They didn't want to be the leaders participating in their state. They were waiting to see what their neighboring hospitals would do. And they did get the bigger hospitals first. So, stating participation in terms of beds, that was a great psychological motivation to those hospitals. . . . But to our managers at the time . . . they looked at their regions and many of them said we have no hospitals participating" (Hess 1991, 11).

Despite the optimistic public relations statistics and confident front, those on the inside of the Title VI compliance effort were getting nervous. Any one of many nightmare scenarios was possible. School desegregation after the *Brown* decision, after all, started out calmly with school districts agreeing to adhere to the law of the land before the backlash and massive resistance set in. Racial civil rights tensions in 1966 were at a fever pitch in many communities. Suppose Governor Wallace made good on his threat to organize southern state resistance? Suppose the Mississippi Sovereignty Commission mounted, with other southern state sovereignty commissions, a skillful, privately funded lobbying and public relations effort as they had done against the Civil Rights Bill, to get hospitals to boycott Medicare and force federal program changes? Suppose someone like Selma's sheriff Jim Clark got the idea to block the entrance of a local small-town hospital with a posse? The local civil rights groups that had served as their undercover allies could also engage in their own protests of lax enforcement, and everything could spin out of control. Suppose black Medicare subscribers were turned away at hospitals that they were now supposed to have a right to access to, and died? During the month of June, all those involved in implementing the Medicare program stayed awake at night worrying about such nightmares.

At the cabinet meeting on June 16, the day after the meeting with hospital leaders, as noted in the White House diary, Johnson asked Deputy Secretary Wilbur Cohen to "investigate the use of federally operated facilities in communities where segregation prevented the operation of Medicare. He asked that the report be given to him by June 18" (White House 1966, 4). The president had, apparently, lost some sleep over the issue as well. The word "segregation" appears nowhere in any public documents as an explanation of these emergency preparations that Johnson's request to Cohen initiated. The Johnson White House maintained tight control over information released by its staff (Berman 1981). Nowhere in any of the public explanations of these preparations is it mentioned that it was a regional problem and related to the persistence of segregation and the refusal to grant Title VI certification to these facilities.

Under Cohen's direction, Robert Ball had organized an emergency taskforce in HEW complete with a situation room. A map of the United States with pins indicated possible trouble spots where a surge in demand might overwhelm local hospitals (Gluck and Reno 2001, 59). The explanation given was that pent-up demand for hospital care would be unleashed by the new Medicare program, but those giving this explanation knew that it was not true. People who need hospital care but can't get it either die or recover on their own—no backlogs develop.[32] Those in the Blue Cross and commercial insurance industry, all acting as consultants to Medicare's implementation and the Social Security Administration's own actuaries knew this. Employers acquiring hospital insurance for their employees knew that use of hospitals grows slowly, not in a rush as if an imaginary dam has broken. Ball acknowledged as much in that a good part of the preparations were to be able to "take action in anticipation of problems under Medicare arising from the application of the Civil Rights Act to hospitals" (Gluck and Reno 2001, 59).

The problem the Medicare program now faced was different from estimating the usual impact of expanded insurance coverage. It is well illustrated by the recollections of one of the Title VI special emissaries. Leon Bernstein, a hospital administrator who had been hired to assist HEW in implementing the program, recalled being sent by Cohen as a special envoy to a hospital near Johnson's birth place in Texas, no doubt at the request of Marvin -Watson in the White House (Bernstein 1976). It had not been certified and would be a political embarrassment to the president. Bernstein met with the hospital's administrator, who was indignant and insisted that they were in full compliance with Title VI. "But you have no black patients even though you have plenty in your service area and you're the only hospital," Bernstein said. "Oh well, they take care of their own," the administrator responded with a shrug (Bernstein 1976). This was the story in many communities—blacks didn't use hospitals except in rare instances and either died or recovered on their own. No one knew at the high-water mark of the civil rights movement what would happen now. Was a real dam about to break?

With Johnson's full support, the emergency Medicare taskforce placed National Guard helicopters on standby and developed plans to transport patients refused admission by local hospitals to military and Veterans Administration facilities. The taskforce convened on June 28 and was, according to the White House diary, to address "hospital compliance with Medicare" (White House 1966, 2). Those participating from HEW were Gardner, Cohen, Stewart, and Lee. Also attending were Attorney General Katzenbach, the assistant secretary of defense, the administrator of Veteran's Affairs, and Douglass Cater, special assistant to the president. About a day later Ted Marmor, an assistant to Wilbur Cohen, recalled being summoned by Marvin Watson to the White House with several other HEW officials. "You tell your boss," Marvin Watson shouted at Marmor, "I don't want any screw-ups, no hitches! You have helicopters ready. I don't want any stories about anyone dying because they were refused hospital care!"[33] Everyone braced for the potential nightmare unraveling of Medicare and the Civil Rights Act.

Johnson conferred briefly with Gardner by phone on June 30 and late that evening talked with Cater, who told him that 94 percent of general hospital beds in the country were now compliant with the civil rights law (White House 1966).

In a televised statement broadcast earlier, Johnson marked the inauguration of the new program: "Medicare begins tomorrow. . . . The program is not just a blessing for older Americans. It is a test for all Americans—a test of our willingness to work together. In the past we have always passed that test. I have no doubt about the future. I believe July 1, 1966 marks a new day of freedom for our people" (L. Johnson 1966c). Certainly OEHO had met the test. Approximately three thousand hospitals had been quietly, uneventfully, and successfully desegregated in less than three months. No National Guard helicopters or backup military hospitals were needed. A key part of national life, one involved in healing our bodies, was now involved in healing our body politic. A social institution that had lagged behind in racial integration was now leading the way. The children's crusade, in spite of the odds, had been victorious.

That victory, however, came with casualties.

5

Casualties

Health care's struggle blended into all the other parts of the larger civil rights struggle. It didn't end with Medicare's triumphal children's crusade any more than the triumphal march from Selma to Montgomery ended the struggle for voting rights. It continued, contested each step of the way, burdened by the loss of the broader optimism that had energized the earlier days of the movement. The Vietnam War, urban riots, white backlash, and growing deficits all added to the discouragement. Change became harder. It involved, to start with, mopping up after early, easier successes.

Mopping Up

On July 1, 1966, the Medicare Program included about sixty-five hundred participating hospitals, 250,000 physicians, twelve hundred home health agencies, seventy-four Blue Cross organizations, thirty-three Blue Shield plans, sixteen insurance companies, and over one hundred prepaid group practices (HMOs) (Ball 1966a, 475). Ninety-seven percent of the short-term general hospital beds in the country were Title VI compliant and participating in the program. In the South, between 200 and 250 hospitals had yet to be certified for compliance. In about one hundred communities in the South less than 75 percent of the beds had been brought into compliance with Title VI, and in a few communities no beds were in compliance, and only emergency admissions to noncompliant hospitals received Medicare payment. (Emergency admissions to nonparticipating hospitals were all concentrated in the South, and it took several years to fully eliminate the use of "emergency" admissions as a way to circumvent Title VI compliance.) While this involved less than 3 percent of the beds, as Social Security commissioner Ball acknowledged, the impact on these communities was serious. "The Public Health Service and I know the American Hospital Association and state associations stand ready to give whatever help we can in bringing about the voluntary compliance of the last 200 or 250 hospitals now not able to participate for civil rights reasons" (Ball 1966a, 476).

Commissioner Ball was also busy responding to complaints and closing loopholes in Title VI enforcement. Complaints to southern senators and congressmen forwarded to Ball from constituents produced prompt, firm, but courteous responses.[1] A constituent complaint sent on June 8, 1966, to Georgia senators Tallmadge and Russell by a recent retiree familiar with his former employer's private insurance coverage was representative:

> Actually only 48 hospitals in Georgia have been cleared to accept Medicare patients on July 1 and it is being intimated that most, if not all large private hospitals in Atlanta may not choose to qualify due to the red tape and the unreasonable attitude of the Federal Government. Two very small hospitals in the Atlanta metropolitan area have been cleared.
>
> The Federal Government has misrepresented Medicare all along by telling us we have a choice of doctor and hospital. This was when they were turning themselves inside out trying to get everybody to sign up for Medical Insurance (Part B). However this is not the case now. They are apparently asking and expecting hospitals to integrate both hospital personnel and their patients—in other words, integration all the way. If a number of hospitals do not choose to qualify then we do not have choice and may not be able to get into a hospital at all that has been certified by the Government. In this event we will have to pay the hospital bill out of our pocket, although at the same time we will be paying Medicare and an insurance company for coverage not covered by Medicare. This is really "taking care" of the "Senior Citizens" if such a condition does exist after July 1, 1966.
>
> I feel Medicare should be amended so that integration and civil rights should have nothing whatever to do with Medicare. Those over 65 can do very little, if anything about civil rights or integration and they should not be made the "Scapegoats" under Medicare. There should not be a lot of red tape in handling a claim under Medicare. I personally handled group insurance claims

with insurance companies for my employer over a period of years with very little difficulty or loss of time. A signed insurance form from the attending doctor and copy of the hospital bill is generally enough to support a claim. If discrimination is involved why not handle it under the civil rights law and not bring civil rights or integration under Medicare, unless the Federal Government just wants to make it difficult for those who signed up for Medicare, as well as for everybody else involved. Frankly, there is not a reason why a hospital should even be approached ahead of time by the Federal Government unless Medicare is going to be used as a "club" for civil rights. . . . It appears the Federal Government is more interested in making this a civil rights and integration deal than they are in taking care of those signed up for Medicare—in spite of their continual promise of "choice of doctor and hospital."

Continually brow-beating the majority may not be a very good way for Democrats to pick up some votes. (Yerkes 1966)

A reply to Senator Russell clarified the law and noted that 87 percent of the beds in Georgia were in compliance and that "some hospitals in Georgia have come into compliance with the civil rights requirements since July 1 and we are hopeful that their example will be followed by the minority of hospitals which have thus far not done so" (Ball 1966b). A similar letter was sent to Representative Hale Boggs (D, LA) in response to a complaint by a lawyer in New Orleans.

Ball would later emphasize the effectiveness and professionalism of local Social Security staff in the South that volunteered for duty in OEHO's Title VI hospital compliance effort as a key to its success. It was not, however, flawless. Ball sent a frosty memo in October 1966 concerning a lapse in assuring Title VI compliance before an agreement with a Mississippi hospital was signed.

On looking into the signing of the agreement with Shelby Hospital in Mississippi, I was disturbed to find that we had not had the report list circulated to the regions and to find that a region had failed to check currently on Title VI status before signing an agreement.

I would like a report on what you plan to do to prevent the reoccurrence of this sort of thing. Unless we can have procedures in the region sufficient to prevent a reoccurrence, it will be necessary to withdraw the delegation from regions that are not properly exercising it and have future agreement from such regions signed centrally after individual central clearance with the Public Health Service. I would hate to have to do this but these occurrences are most embarrassing to the Social Security Administration and cannot be allowed to continue.

On the whole it seems to me that an excellent job has been done in securing compliance with Title VI and we do not want the record marred at the end of the process. (Ball 1966c)

Whoever was responsible for this lapse, it is not likely that it happened again.

The White House, without any interference, allowed the HEW group to proceed with the mopping up process, which included administrative appeals from some resistant southern hospitals searching for a weakness they could exploit. Johnson continued to worry about a backlash and was especially attentive to news coverage. On the CBS evening news Daniel Schorr aired a story about a Mississippi hospital that was discharging all their elderly patients as a result of their refusal to comply with Medicare's Title VI requirements. Wilbur Cohen told Libassi he was going to be interviewed by Schorr in a follow-up and to "give him our side of the story." The day after Schorr's follow-up interview, Cohen called Libassi to his office and gave him an enthusiastic hug. "I was with the President discussing the education programs with Gardner and Howe (Commissioner of Education). Johnson stopped and turned on the Schorr TV interview with you. I was so glad about how well you handled it. I would have had hell to pay if you had messed up. As it was, we just went back to talking about the education programs without a single pause!"[2] By January 1967 the mopping up, with only a few exceptions, had been completed.

One of the loose ends that took a more time to tie up, however, involved racially segregated state psychiatric hospitals. Psychiatric hospitals remained a state responsibility and did not receive federal funds from Medicare or Medicaid. They were, however, public facilities and still received federal funds for construction, training, and research. OEHO began to investigate them shortly after the implementation of the Medicare program. The fate of these facilities and the consequences in the aftermath of the Civil Rights Act deserves book-length treatment all by itself. Suffice it here to say that, faced with the threat of loss of federal funds, only three states, Virginia, Mississippi, and Alabama, put up a fight. These states argued that they didn't segregate patients by race because they allowed them "freedom of choice." For those in OEHO involved in negotiating with these states, the argument was even more absurd than it had been in forcing desegregation of the acute care general hospitals.

> The "freedom of choice" issue was to us quite bizarre, even as applied to patients in general hospitals. In those cases, as related by a black witness in one of the early hearings, who testified that he did not "choose" that his daughter be placed in the white wing of the hospital (or double room with a white patient) because of the risks taken by such a choice. As he suggested, "who knows what would be done to her in the hospital after I would make such a choice." To us, in a mental hospital, it was even more ridiculous—people were being confined in these institutions because they lacked the capacity to make rational choices. (Rose 1997, 3)

The first state psychiatric hospital system OEHO took on was in Virginia, beginning in the fall of 1966. Virginia had one state hospital for blacks and three for whites and argued that a "freedom of choice" system it had put in place did not violate Title VI requirements. The state was given a notice of hearing, and Nash, at a meeting with the University of Virginia psychiatry department, had given them the impression, albeit incorrect, that their own federal funding would be jeopardy. This had led to the intervention of the governor, who was more than happy to use such an excuse, however incorrect, to end the "freedom of choice" deception. Not everyone in the state government was willing to go along, and the assistant attorney general assigned to handling the signing of the settlement in Richmond in December 1966 angrily compared it to "Appomattox" (Rose 1997, 5).

Altogether, about three hundred acute care general hospitals were still awaiting clearance for Title VI on July 1, 1966, and about another three hundred had chosen to not to apply and remain segregated. As many as two dozen others that had received initial clearance were subsequently sent notices of hearings to revoke their Title VI certification (see, for example, Bell 1966). With a few exceptions, all but those that had chosen to remain outside of the Medicare program were resolved by the end of 1966. The nonparticipating hospitals that otherwise could have qualified tended to be well-endowed institutions that did so as a matter of principle and often out of an inflated sense of their own self-importance. Most were certain that they would be able to wait out the feds and get the Medicare dollars on their own terms. One of the last of these to comply with Title VI requirements was Baptist Hospital in Jackson, Mississippi. St. Dominic's, the Catholic hospital in the city, had chosen to comply. Baptist's board and medical staff watched with frustration as St. Dominic's hospital market share expanded and its own financial position deteriorated. In 1969, St. Dominic's broke ground on a new addition that would double its beds to more than four hundred. Finally, in a nine-to-four vote on April 9, 1969, the board of Baptist Hospital voted to begin talking to federal officials about what would be required to be certified for Medicare funds (*Clarion Ledger* 1969). By the end of the year all the hospitals in Jackson, the epicenter of resistance to integration, were officially integrated. It had been the domestic equivalent of the Cold War struggle. It was not without casualties, and the war wasn't over.

The Fallen

Maya Lin's Civil Rights Memorial in Montgomery, Alabama, is a few blocks from the White House of the Confederacy and a block from Dexter Avenue Baptist Church, where Martin Luther King helped begin the bus boycott. Just like her Vietnam War Memorial in Washington, it lists the names of the fallen. Water flows over the forty-one names listed, and its inscription reads, "Until justice rolls down like waters and righteousness like a mighty stream" (Amos 5:24). The list begins with those connected to T. R. M. Howard and the Regional Council of Negro Leadership, murdered in Mississippi in 1955, and ends with Martin Luther King's assassination in Memphis in 1968. This narrow band of time implies a beginning and an end, a brief anomaly unconnected to the nation's past and present. Yet there were no such insulating boundaries in health care or any other of the interrelated parts of that larger struggle. The deaths of three individuals illustrate this, one for each stage of the much longer health care and larger civil rights struggle. James Chaney died in the midst of the struggle for voting rights in Jackson, Mississippi, and the efforts to desegregate the state's major teaching hospital. Jean Cowsert died in Mobile, Alabama, in the midst of a struggle to extend Title VI hospital accountability to its medical staff and a growing backlash against civil rights efforts. Fred Hampton died in Chicago, Illinois, in the midst of struggle with police and an effort to provide access to the poor to basic primary care in the bitter, contested aftermath of the civil rights era.

JAMES CHANEY

Jackson, Mississippi, and its hospitals had been at the epicenter of the South's civil rights struggle. The bodies of James Chaney, Michael Schwerner, and Andrew Goodman were found beneath an earthen dam near Philadelphia, Mississippi, on August 4, 1964. The FBI ordered them taken to the University of Mississippi Medical Center in Jackson, and they arrived just after midnight on August 5. Three pathologists on the staff of the medical center did the autopsies. No information was released at the request of the FBI, and the bureau's statement to the press simply reported that the three had been shot. At the request of the parents of Chaney and Schwerner, independent autopsies were performed by Dr. David Spain, a pathologist from the Brookdale Medical Center in New York. His account of Chaney's autopsy, published in *Ramparts*, was later incorporated into a lecture by Louis Lasagna, MD, reproduced in the *Yale Journal of Biology and Medicine*.

> One of the University's pathologists stepped forward, silently, and helped me slide Chaney's corpse . . . to the stainless steel examining table in the middle of the room. He stepped backward and lined up with his three comrades on one side of the table facing me. The only sound in the green-tiled room was the rough noise of the zipper of the protective plastic bag as I pulled it away from Chaney's body. I was immediately struck by how slight and frail the young man was— . . . I couldn't find the bullet hole (in the wrist) the newspapers mentioned. The wrist was broken all right. Bones were smashed, so badly that his wrist must have been literally flapping when he was carried. But there was no indication of any bullet hole. I looked up at the three doctors opposite me. Their faces were stone. I motioned to the wrist. I asked where the bullet hole was. One of the stone figures facing me offered a mumbled explanation something about how Chaney's hand had been across his chest when the first examination was made and the examiner must have mistaken the bullet hole in the chest for the one in the hand. I looked at him in amazement. Then I noticed Chaney's jaw. It was

broken—the lower jaw was completely shattered, split vertically, by some tremendous force. I moved the shattered pieces of his jaw in the vertical direction for the three doctors to see. They remained silent. I couldn't catch their eyes. I carefully examined the body, and found that the bones in the right shoulder were crushed—again from some strong and direct blow. . . . One thing was certain: this frail boy had been beaten in an inhuman fashion. . . . I surmised he must have been beaten with chains or a pipe. . . . It was impossible to say if he had died before he was shot. . . . I examined his skull and it was crushed, too. I could barely believe the destruction to these frail young bones. In my twenty-five years as a pathologist and medical examiner, I have never seen bones so severely shattered, except in tremendously high speed accidents or airplane crashes.

It was obvious to any first-year medical student that the boy had been beaten to a pulp. I have been conducting examinations of this type for a quarter of a century, but for the first time I found myself so emotionally charged that it was difficult to retain my professional composure. I felt like screaming at these impassive observers still silent standing across the table. But I knew that no rage of mine would tear the curtain of silence. I took off my green surgical smock . . . and left the room as fast as I could. (Lasagna 1965b, 362–63)

Director of the medical center Robert Marston, MD, was quick to come to the defense of his colleagues, and his letter was published in a subsequent issue of the *Yale Journal of Biology and Medicine*. He quoted several letters from J. Edgar Hoover thanking the pathologists for their assistance in the investigation and concludes, "I trust these sober and forthright statements of the cooperativeness and effectiveness of our department in aiding the FBI in obtaining full and complete information will serve to correct the unwarranted false implications made in this regard" (Marston 1965, 47). His defense of an aggressive policy of not releasing any information does not stand up well in the light of subsequent revelations of FBI misconduct in the handling of civil rights activists nor to any standard of decency in the treatment of the families of the victims. Lasagna noted in his response to Marston's protest, "Nothing would please me more than to learn that any and all Mississippi physicians were completely innocent of distorting the truth. Perhaps one day the complete story will be told" (Lasagna 1965a, 47).

Paul Johnson, governor of Mississippi at the time, reported his version of the story later in an interview:

> Actually, one thing that is not known to people anywhere in this country is that these Klansmen—of course I knew them well; most of them supported me when I ran for governor— . . . did not actually intend to kill these people. What happened was that they had been taken from jail and brought to this particular spot. There were a good many people in the group besides the sheriff and the deputy sheriff and that group. What they were going to do, they were going to hang these three persons in a big cotton sack and leave them hanging in the tree for about a day or a day and a half, then come out there at night and turn them loose. They thought that they'd more or less scare them off. While they were talking this Negro boy from over in Meridian (James Chaney), he seemed like the ringleader of the three—He was acting kind of smart aleck and talking pretty big, and one of the Klansman walked up behind him and hit him over the head with a trace chain you use, as you know, (for) plowing and that sort of thing. And the end of a trace chain as you know, is about that large [two or three inches]. . . . The chain came across his head and hit him just above the bridge of the nose and killed him dead as a nit. After this boy had been killed, then is when they determined, "Well, we got to dispose of the other two." (P. Johnson 1970, 32–33)

A month before James Chaney's autopsy, the Civil Rights Act of 1964 became law. Marston and the University of Mississippi Medical center, if for no other reason than the lure of the federal dollars that would enable it to flourish, were on the way "without unnecessary delay or unworkable haste" to comply (Quinn 2005, 85).

DR. JEAN COWSERT

Dr. Jean Cowsert returned to Mobile from the meeting at the White House where President Johnson made his final plea for compliance with Title VI on June 15, 1966. It was uncertain which, if any, Mobile facilities would be cleared for participation in the Medicare program. The 327 hospitals still awaiting Title VI clearance on June 30, 1966, included all four of Mobile's. Indeed, Mobile had become the center of a bitter, clandestine, high-stakes battle that would determine how substantial the changes brought by the Title VI enforcement effort would be. Unknown to any of the local combatants, Jean Cowsert was in the middle of it.

Up until 1965, hospital care in Mobile had been rigidly separate and far from equal. The 540-bed Mobile Infirmary, the well-endowed, dominant institution in the region's social and medical hierarchy, served whites only. Mobile General, the 247-bed county facility serving the indigent, had racially segregated accommodations, as did Providence Hospital, a 262-bed facility operated by the Daughters of Charity of St. Vincent de Paul. A thirty-five-bed private black hospital, St. Martin de Porres, the only hospital where black physicians could get staff privileges, had been established in the 1950s as a token concession to the separate but equal requirements of the Hill-Burton Act.

All four of the hospitals in Mobile had received Hill-Burton funding for construction. After the passage of the 1964 Civil Rights Act, just as in other communities, the segregated pattern of care in these hospitals had been challenged by a local civil rights group. The Nonpartisan Voters League (the NAACP had been outlawed in Alabama) had submitted complaints to James Quigley, HEW assistant secretary responsible for civil rights. It was also working with the NAACP Legal Defense Fund to bring suits against the hospitals.

Dr. Cowsert was apparently drawn into these struggles by institutional loyalty, personal friendship, and her own fierce independence as a medical practitioner. A native of Mobile, she served in the Army Signal Corps as a radio and radar technician during World War II. She went on to graduate at the top of her medical school class at the University of Alabama in 1954, one of two women in a class of sixty-two. Dr. Cowsert and five other women who graduated at the top of their medical school classes in the United State that year received American Medical Woman's Association awards of achievement at an event in Chicago. (A wire service story tried to soften this threat to 1950s sensibilities by pointing out that "not only did they top the men in class—some of them balanced long study hours with baby-raising, dishwashing and cooking for a husband" [INS 1955].) After an internship and residency in Detroit, Michigan, she returned to Mobile in 1959 to set up her internal medicine practice.

Her primary hospital affiliation was with Providence, a 262-bed facility operated by the Daughters of Charity of St. Vincent de Paul. She had become friends with its administrator, Sister Andrea Hickey, and some of the other nuns connected to the hospital, and she was in the process of converting to Catholicism. Dr. Cowsert served as chief of medical services between 1962 and 1963, the first woman in the history of any of the hospitals in Mobile to serve in this capacity. She had been instrumental in getting Providence to become a participant in the Professional Activity Study (PAS), an early effort to review the admission practices and quality of care of medical staff members through computerized discharge abstracts. Providence was the first hospital in Alabama to participate in PAS, making it a pioneer in hospital monitoring of care, still resisted by most hospital medical staffs and yet to be established as a clear legal responsibility for hospitals.

In 1965, Providence Hospital also broke ranks with the other hospitals in Mobile and desegregated. The religious order, based in St. Louis, Missouri, did not face the resistance to integration that local community boards imposed on the other hospitals in town. In recognition of its efforts to integrate, the Non-partisan Voters League notified HEW's James Quigley on August 13, 1965, that it was withdrawing its earlier complaint against the hospital. "We are pleased to advise you that Providence Hospital now projects a picture which indicates that it is in compliance with Title VI of the Civil Rights Act. The hospital, in our opinion, has pursued a determined policy in almost all areas to meet the demands of Title VI" (Leflore 1965a). Providence, however, had paid a heavy price for this decision. A nurse who had been employed at Providence during this period noted,

> It was a difficult transition for everybody. Many white patients
> refused admission and went to the Mobile Infirmary instead.
> The census dropped way down. The administrator and some of
> the nurses from the North were resented. Whites that did come
> sometimes brought their own pillows so they wouldn't have to sleep
> on the ones blacks had. Many would try to change rooms or move
> into a private one if they had to share one with a black patient. We
> were an older facility and had few private rooms to accommodate
> such transfers. The blacks didn't like the change either.[3]

In essence, Providence demonstrated why voluntary desegregation never worked and why federal universally imposed desegregation was the only way to do it. Providence, at least from the perspective of Dr. Cowsert, was being punished for obeying the law and the Infirmary rewarded for breaking it. Perhaps not wishing to exacerbate Providence's problems and hoping that all the hospitals in Mobile could be brought into compliance before the deadline, OEHO held off signing off on Title VI compliance for any of Mobile's hospitals. On July 1, 1966, however, Providence, Mobile General, and St. Martin de Porres received Title VI approval. The Mobile Infirmary, the largest and most influential hospital in the region, did not.

Not clearing the Mobile Infirmary was a risky, high-stakes gamble for OEHO. It moved OEHO into trying to address for the first time the explosive unresolved issue of a hospital's responsibilities for the discriminatory admission practices of its medical staff. A hospital could, in theory, do everything it was required to do to comply with Title VI and yet remain completely segregated simply as a result of the discriminatory decisions of medical staff members about where they would admit their patients of different races. This appeared to be what was happening at the Mobile Infirmary. If hospitals could do what the Mobile Infirmary appeared to be doing it could undermine the entire Title VI compliance effort.

OEHO decided to use the Mobile Infirmary to try to find a way to address the major flaw in the Title VI enforcement effort. HEW had chosen to exempt physicians from compliance with Title VI. Part B of Medicare, the part reimbursing for physician services, it argued, was a form of federal assistance in the way of a "contract of insurance or guaranty." The Civil Rights Act had exempted such federal assistance from Title VI. The exclusion assured that Title VI would not be used to attack housing discrimination by blocking any use of federally insured mortgages and bank deposits in any way related to racially discriminatory housing. Fair housing legislation soon eliminated this loophole (Title VIII of the Civil Rights Act of 1968, passed a week after the assassination of Martin Luther King), but no legislation has ever overturned HEW's decision to exempt Part B of Medicare. In theory, physicians could keep their segregated waiting rooms and still receive Medicare reimbursement. This exemption, however, helped assure physician participation in Medicare and freed HEW from trying to figure out how it could possibly enforce Title VI in the more hidden world of private medical practice.

A combination of the cumulative complaints against the Mobile Infirmary and the hospital's intransigence made confrontation inevitable. During the last six months of 1965, in a hospital service area that was

33 percent black, only ten of the almost ten thousand patients admitted to the Infirmary had been black. A deposition collected by the Nonpartisan Voters League suggests that that those blacks that had been admitted may have been the result of "errors" by their admitting physicians and had to overcome many hurdles imposed by the hospital's admission process:

On May 21, 1965 my wife, Willie Mae Myles, was admitted to the Mobile Infirmary for the birth of our child. Dr. Norton, the physician who treated my wife, asked her what hospital she wanted to go to. My wife asked what hospital did he recommend and he said the Mobile Infirmary because you can get better service there and at the same cost. My wife is real fair or light skinned complexion and the doctor evidently thought she was a white person. When it was time for the baby to be born I carried Willie May to the Mobile Infirmary. After arriving at the hospital we went into the office where three white ladies were admitting patients. They could easily determine that I was Negro. One of the ladies asked, "What doctor sent you here?" I told the name of the doctor. She asked, "Which Dr. Norton?" They wanted to transfer her to Mobile General and offered to pay for an ambulance to transfer her. I refused to accept the offer and reminded them that I thought the Civil Rights Act should protect my wife in this matter. I told them, "I have paid the doctor and he sent Willie Mae here and I am not going to take her any other place." The lady asked, "Do you have insurance?" I said, "Yes," and I showed her my hospital insurance papers from the Independence Insurance Company. The lady said, "I cannot take this insurance." I was then sent to the main office. I sat in the office about twenty minutes and a Mr. Booth, Assistant Director of the Mobile Infirmary came to talk to me. Mr. Booth, asked, who sent your wife to the Infirmary?" I told him, "Dr. Norton, the physician treating her recommended this hospital." He then asked about hospital insurance. I showed him the same insurance papers that I had previously showed the lady in the admittance office. He then said, "We cannot accept this type of insurance because it against the rules of the staff." . . . I asked, "If this is a segregated hospital." He said, "I wouldn't say that but your wife will be the first colored woman admitted for childbirth." Mr. Booth told me that I would have to get $100 for an admittance fee. I told him that I didn't have $100 at the moment. I further said that after my wife had the baby and is discharged, I would pay the balance of the bill that will not be covered by insurance. Mr. Booth did finally take the insurance papers. (Non-partisan Voters' League 1965)

Indeed, the deposition suggests, at least for the Mobile Infirmary, the joke about the Chicago voluntary hospitals where black births were "smuggled into the hospital in the wombs of white mothers" had some truth to it. Yet the Infirmary had signed all the compliance forms and insisted that they had admitted every patient referred to them by their medical staff regardless of race. Nevertheless, they refused to provide any the statistics on the admissions of individual physicians and refused to intervene in any way in the admission decisions of their medical staff, insisting that it was a private decision made by the doctor and his patient. In the meantime, J. L. Leflore, head of the Non-partisan Voters League, sent a letter to Quigley:

Confidential but reliable informants accuse the Director of the Hospital and leaders of its medical staff of working clandestinely to avoid complying with the civil rights act. We understand that those responsible for policy at the Mobile Infirmary are desperately but suavely defying the law relative to the acceptance of Negro patients and the integration of its medical staff and personnel, other than on a token basis. There are those in knowledge of the hospital situation in Mobile who cannot feel it merely accidental that 15 to 18% of patients accepted to Providence hospital are Negro and that the 527 bed Mobile Infirmary had only 15 Negro patients since our petition was filed on March 24, 1965. (Leflore 1965b)

All the hospitals in Mobile were a few blocks from each other, and most physicians had multiple hospital privileges. This permitted physicians, without wasting travel time, to see their white patients in the white hospital, their black patients in the black hospital, their indigent patients in the public hospital, and their Catholic patients in the Catholic hospital. Pressures on physicians to admit "the right kind" of patients to a particular hospital was not unique to southern cities. Chicago, for example, had maintained a high degree of segregation in hospital care simply through the choices of physicians about where they would admit their patients. Custom dictated where you sent which patients, and physicians were often concerned that if they did too much to buck such customs they might not get their privileges renewed.

In the case of the Mobile Infirmary, many medical staff members had apparently pledged at a medical staff meeting never to admit any of their black patients to the Infirmary. The "confidential informant" who had pointed this out and who had later provided a list of the coconspirators that was forwarded to the OEHO was Dr. Jean Cowsert. As a Mobile Infirmary medical staff member who attended their meetings, she now served as OEHO's "mole." She volunteered for this duty either before or shortly after her attendance at Johnson's White House Conference. Her participation was key to the decision to try to use the Mobile Infirmary as a test case for insisting that a hospital had a responsibility for assuring that the admission practices of its medical staff complied with Title VI requirements.

The refusal to sign off on the Infirmary's Title VI compliance became a bitter test of wills. The Infirmary insisted that it had complied with all the requirements, refused to release any information on the admissions patterns of individual staff members, and did whatever it could to circumvent OEHO and its exclusion from the Medicare program. Medicare allowed for the payment for admissions to non-participating hospitals in the case of emergencies. All the Medicare admissions to the infirmary after July 1, 1966, were defined as "emergencies." Cowsert apparently alerted OEHO staff of this subterfuge, and these payments were stopped. As a result, the census in the Mobile Infirmary dropped, and an entire wing with one hundred beds was shut down. Negotiations with the OEHO staff and the hospital remained at an impasse. By December, pressure had built up to the point that top HEW officials tried to intervene to end the stalemate. Marilyn Rose, who served as legal counsel to OEHO and its director, Robert Nash, recalls the rest of the story:

> All hell broke loose in terms of political pressure. There was
> extensive daily media coverage in Alabama and intense pressure
> was put on HEW. . . . Bob Nash, Rose Brock and I met with Dr. Leo
> Gehrig (Assistant Surgeon General of the Public Health Service)
> who was being sent to Mobile to meet with hospital officials and

other people in the community. . . . Gehrig wanted to be filled in on particulars. In addition to the obvious discussion of the admission particulars Gehrig was given sources of information which was not a matter of public record. This information included the name and the telephone number of a woman physician on the hospital staff who gave OEHO inside information, including clear instances of racist statements and defiant attitudes of staff physicians at staff meetings on the admission practices of the hospital. . . . Either Bob Nash or Rose Brock advised Leo Gehrig to contact her for current information. It was clear that her identity needed to be kept a secret as she would be looked at as a traitor if her identity would be revealed.

Gehrig came back with great enthusiasm, and a plan which he described at a meeting to Nash, Brock and me. We thought that the plan would not work . . . and was just another stall.

At that meeting Gehrig also related that he talked with the woman physician, and, in the course of that aspect of the report we learned that he had talked to her in a telephone conversation he had made from his hotel room. . . . We never called anyone in such circumstances from any phone other than one in a phone booth, and not the same phone as previous phone calls. (In those days civil rights workers generally understood that phones were tapped. While we could not guarantee that the recipient's phone was not tapped, we took great effort to protect our end of the call.)

Ten days later, at about seven in the morning, Bob Nash got a telephone call from the Administrator of the Mobile Infirmary advising him that this woman had been "accidentally" shot to death. . . . She was found outside her home, in her bathrobe, a stone had apparently been thrown through her window and she appeared to have gone out with her gun to investigate. The coroner's report was that she was accidentally shot, apparently having tripped, and shot herself. To this day I do not believe that finding. It seems just too coincidental. What led the hospital administrator to call Nash about this incident, unless the word had gotten out that she was an informer . . . if he knew she was an informer, others knew, and the knowledge may very well have come from the telephone call through the hotel switchboard. . . . The referral practices issue was dead after the Mobile cave in. (Rose 1997, 12–14)

In other words, the effort to test whether OEHO could extend a hospital's Title VI responsibilities to the admission practices of its medical staff had failed. A few days after Dr. Cowsert's death, on January 27, 1967, the Mobile Infirmary received "provisional" Title VI clearance retroactive to February 1, 1967. There had been some modest improvement in admission statistics. "Medicare Fight Won by Hospital," a *Mobile Register* headline read (*Mobile Register* 1967). On June 28, 1967, the home of J. L. Leflore, who had led the local civil rights movement effort to desegregate Mobile's hospitals, was firebombed. On July 1, 1967, the Mobile Infirmary received full Title VI clearance. Six months later the Mobile Infirmary census reached 93 percent, and it was completing plans for a six story addition (Smith 2009, 42).

The pathologist employed by the Mobile Infirmary, Dr. Earl Wert, served as coroner at the time. It was a job that paid $100 a month and had been previously filled by funeral directors. There was nothing in terms of equipment. He didn't remember the examination of Dr. Cowsert but acknowledged the limitations of the resources available to him in conducting a thorough investigation. Dr. Wert recalled her as being a strong and abrasive person who didn't get along with the other doctors and was not a part of the group of physicians in Mobile that worked and socialized together. "Providence at that time was for the have-nots and the Infirmary was for the haves, so I can imagine how she felt."[4]

The Mobile Infirmary's administrator, E. C. Bramlett Sr., acknowledged the problem of doctors refusing to admit black patients to the Infirmary but insisted the Infirmary kept with their own plan for gradual integration and prevailed (Harriman 2011, 181–97). Indeed, today the percentage of black Medicare admissions to the Mobile Infirmary roughly matches its percentage of the population in the Mobile metropolitan area. The Mobile Infirmary, as other hospitals in the area, converted to all single-bed rooms, circumventing any problems with room assignment by race. E. C. Bramlett Jr. (part of a family dynasty of administrators operating the Infirmary through most of the twentieth century), recalling the hospital's history during this period, insisted that it was "fully integrated" and the only trouble it had was with the White Citizens' Councils, which wanted to keep the Mobile Infirmary white only. He blamed the withholding of Title VI approval on the federal "zealots" who wanted to do away with the private practice of medicine. The hospital had no control over the admitting practices of its medical staff who admitted people where they felt most comfortable, and it was not going to kick anyone off its medical staff on that basis. "It took almost an act of Congress to overturn the HEW decision."[5]

The mystery of Jean Cowsert's death, as well as a hospital's broader social accountability for its medical staff members' admission practices, remains unresolved. No records of the autopsy, police investigation, alleged FBI investigation, or correspondence during this period between the hospital and their congressman or with the OEHO now exists, and events surrounding her death have disappeared from local memory.[6] While studies continue to document racial disparities in admission patterns for specialty care, no comparable challenge, expanding a hospital's responsibility in this area, has since been mounted.

It took amazing backbone for Jean Cowsert to do what she did. Her death was a tragic loss to medicine and the movement for social justice. One could not possibly turn her story into fiction because it would not be believable. In the words of Garrison Keeler's detective Guy Noir, who must have been thinking about Mobile, "It's a dark night in a city that knows how to keep its secrets."

FRED HAMPTON

Fred Hampton graduated from high school in the Chicago suburb of Maywood in 1966, just as Chicago was becoming the national focus of the civil rights efforts. A coalition of local civil rights groups that included the NAACP and the Coordinating Council of Community Organizations (CCCO) had brought the Title VI complaint against the Chicago schools. They had been demoralized by the White House's decision in the fall of 1965 to override the commissioner of education and release the Elementary and Secondary Education Act funding to Chicago. It needed star power to reenergize their grass roots protests and looked to Martin Luther King and the SCLC, fresh from their march from Selma to Montgomery and their Voting Rights Act triumph, to provide it. King and the SCLC were also at a critical turning point. The visible color lines enforced by Jim Crow laws were coming down. The more intractable, invisible ones in northern cities had to be the next target of the movement. Chicago seemed to offer the three key ingredients that could, at least in terms of moral symbolism, turn the tide in this new stage of the civil rights struggle: (1) abysmal conditions in Chicago's South and West Side ghettos, (2) active local civil rights groups, and (3) the potential for a vivid, visual moral confrontation similar to that provided by Sherriff Jim Clark in Selma and Bull Connor in Birmingham. Chicago, as King and SCLC would discover to their dismay, offered too much of all three. Hampton had begun a prelaw program at a junior college while working as a youth organizer for the NAACP. He was soon drawn into the resulting maelstrom.[7]

In the same year of Fred Hampton's high school graduation the hospitals in Chicago had swiftly passed Title VI inspections for Medicare funds. The Title VI debacle with Mayor Daly and the Chicago schools appeared to have had a spillover effect, making the Title VI certification of Chicago's hospitals more pro forma than was perhaps warranted. The Committee to End Discrimination in Chicago's Medical Institutions in 1966 submitted a Title VI complaint against the city's hospitals. They reworked and updated the birth and death statistics for Chicago's hospitals showing that little had changed.[8] It asked OEHO to block the release of Medicare funds to all the hospitals in Chicago until the problem was acknowledged and addressed. Such an action would have certainly gotten the attention of the Chicago medical community. Yet, with the Johnson administration's Chicago School Board cave-in fresh in its mind, HEW was probably not eager to get burned again. OEHO's fourteen-person team quickly surveyed all the hospitals in the area. According to the head of the effort, Dr. Fredrick Plotke, it "found no complaints of discrimination that could be substantiated," and its team had been "cordially welcomed at all the institutions and found no instance of overt discrimination" (*Chicago Daily Defender* 1966). Dr. Leonidas Berry, a physician practicing at Cook County, president of the local NMA chapter, and a complaint participant, noted that the difference in their positions hinged on the word "overt." He also noted that the "first meeting between local authorities and Negro doctors came after all the big hospitals in town had already been given a clean bill of health on practices regarding race relations. . . . If there is compliance, then that compliance is only superficial, and I deplore what has happened" (*Chicago Daily Defender* 1966).

In fairness, unlike Chicago's schools, which were accountable to a single superintendent and board, Chicago's hospitals were independent entities, and the veil of innocence was even more tightly drawn. It would have been hard to hold each accountable for the de facto segregation in the hospital system as whole. Chicago's hospitals, even more than its school system, could argue that they were just the victims of larger social and demographic forces beyond their control. Indeed, the guidelines for Title VI compliance distributed to hospitals by the Public Health Service make no mention of the subtle forms of unequal treatment reflected in the overall patterns of hospital use in Chicago. It is, however, telling that, unlike the typical procedure in southern communities of meeting with black leaders and physicians in preparation for hospital inspections, the contact in Chicago with such individuals came only after the certification of all the major medical centers had been completed.

The CCCO-SCLC partnership, the Chicago Freedom Movement (CFM), coalesced around an agenda during the summer of 1966. Hampton, a foot soldier in the campaign but a bright student of politics and a charismatic speaker, soon came to the attention of its leadership. He recruited more than five hundred teens to the NAACP youth movement for the CFM protests. That campaign shaped him and everything that would follow in his life.

The CFM chose to launch their attack against housing discrimination in Chicago. It was concrete and central to addressing all the problems of racial injustice in Chicago. The resulting demonstrations were greeted with racial taunts and violence in neighborhoods that matched anything that had happened previously in southern protests. King would later acknowledge, "I have never seen such hostility and hatred anywhere in my life, even in Selma" (qtd. in Anderson and Pickering 1986, 228). Yet the police, unlike in Selma, took their share of abuse protecting the demonstrators. A tense series of summit meetings with city leadership in August 1966 succeeded in briefly ending the demonstrations but nothing that satisfied the demonstrators. Just forcing expansion of the boundaries of the black ghetto didn't solve the housing segregation problem. It was unclear what would.

The November 1966 elections marked cold new realities for the Chicago Freedom Movement and the national civil rights struggle, which had already started to ebb. Overall, Republicans gained forty-seven seats in the House and three in the Senate. In Illinois, Republican Charles Percy replaced longtime civil rights supporter Senator Paul Douglas. Illinois's other senator, Everett Dirksen, who had supported the Civil Rights Act of 1964, voted against the 1966 Civil Rights Bill because of its open housing provisions. The bill failed to pass. It would seem unfair to call these results a civil rights "backlash" any more than the hostile receptions Chicago marches received in white neighborhoods. That would imply that the movement caused it. Rather, it was a realization of how much self-interest was tied up in the status quo and how difficult the struggle for real change would be. The participants in the CFM open housing campaign had all concluded by December that nothing had changed. Division in the movement over leadership, local tactics, black power, and the Vietnam War fragmented the movement and further weakened it. In April 1967, Daly had won reelection by a large majority, and King had begun to disengage from the Chicago effort. The Chicago Freedom Movement faded away.

A year later, on April 3, 1968, King's assassination in Memphis triggered riots in Chicago and in about one hundred other cities. The riots in Chicago were worse than any since 1919. Concentrated mostly on the West Side, rioters moved from block to block breaking store windows and looting. Fires raged out of control. Altogether about 10,500 police, 6,700 Illinois National Guard troops, and 5,000 US Army soldiers were assigned to quell the disturbances. The riots left eleven citizens dead, forty-eight wounded, ninety policemen injured, and 2,150 people arrested. Two miles of Lawndale on West Madison Street on the West Side were left in rubble. The riot was then more than matched by the rhetoric and finger pointing that followed. The nation seemed on the verge of violent disintegration.

In the wake of the West Side riot, Fred Hampton and the Black Panther Party emerged from the rubble. It was a new form of activism that viewed nonviolence as just one of many tactics in what Hampton regarded as a class struggle. The West Side's residents were mostly more recent migrants from the Deep South who had been pushed out of Chicago's South Side by urban renewal. The Panthers' community self-help and self-defense approach seemed to reflect more the traditional southern rural culture of the West Side residents than the Panthers' Maoist rhetoric, but it was the rhetoric that got the attention of the Chicago police and the FBI.

Hampton soon became its chairman. Over the next year Hampton formed a "rainbow coalition" (a name and political strategy that Jessie Jackson and later Barack Obama subsequently appropriated). That coalition grew to include the Blackstone Rangers (a black South Side youth gang that had gotten involved in the CFM), the Young Patriots (an uptown poor white Appalachian youth gang), the Young Lords (a Puerto Rican gang), the Brown Berets (a Chicano group), and the Students for Democratic Society (SDS—having a white, college-educated membership). It was an odd collection of alliances that combined those with a history of gang violence and criminal activity and those with left-wing political causes.

The Chicago Black Panthers had a concrete action program, which they exported to some of the other groups in their emerging rainbow coalition. The Panthers saw their mission as "serving the people." They set up free breakfast programs for kids and clinics for the community. They babysat children and helped the elderly with their groceries, as well as showing blatant disrespect for the police, who functioned as a hostile occupying force on the West Side. The Panthers, on the balance, reflected a fresh community spirit that attracted recruits the same way that socially concerned individuals are attracted to the ministry and to the police force (Rice 1998, 73).

In July 1969, a Panthers spokesperson announced that they would open a free medical clinic "to serve the needs of all oppressed peoples. The people need a medical program run without any red tape; one that gives services simply because people need it" (*Chicago Daily Defender* 1969). The Panther spirit of inclusive radicalism drew many white volunteers to its efforts, including Chicago medical students shaped by the 1960s counterculture to help staff its free clinic. That sometimes required corrections to fit with the more disciplined Black Panther view of its mission, as Quentin Young, one of the Medical Committee for Human Rights volunteers, described later:

> The Black Panther Clinic was a classy place to be. It enjoyed significant support among medical students. All the kids at the clinic were counterculture, antiwar and dressed grungy. They used to give me a hard time because I dressed in a tie and a suit. I had enough problems and didn't want to make a statement with my clothes. One day the director (Ronald "Doc" Satchell) of the Black Panther Clinic called everyone into the recreation room for a special meeting. "You are confusing the people," he announced to the group. "From now on I want you all to put on a shirt and a tie and dress like physicians."[9]

Shortly after the opening of the clinic, J. Edgar Hoover's FBI COINTELPRO, an extralegal program designed to undermine radical political groups and particularly black civil rights groups, focused its campaign in Chicago against the Panthers and more specifically on Fred Hampton. According to Hoover, the Panthers were a "violence prone organization seeking to overthrow the Government by revolutionary means" and the nation's "number one threat to internal security" (qtd. in Nelson 2011, 146). It was a baffling assessment even for the agents involved in monitoring its activities. Nevertheless, Hoover directed the COINTELPRO to "neutralize the Black Panther Party and destroy what the BPP stands for" and "eradicate its 'serve the people' programs" (qtd. in Nelson 2011, 146). That had resulted in an FBI raid, three Chicago police raids on the Panthers, and other efforts to disrupt and discredit them. The last of these raids, while Hampton was out of town, resulted in the death of two police officers and a nineteen-year-old Panther, Spurgeon Winter Jr. In a move not designed to reduce any of the enmity between the Panthers and the Chicago police, the Panthers' clinic was renamed in his honor. A fourth raid, described by a local community member as a "Northern lynching," targeted Hampton (qtd. in Haas 2009, 89). If anything, it was more chilling than the Klan killing of James Chaney and the other two civil rights workers in Mississippi five years earlier.

The FBI provided artful planning for the raid. A paid FBI informant, William O'Neal, had infiltrated the Panthers, befriended Hampton, served as his bodyguard, and tried to entrap younger Panthers in criminal activities. O'Neal supplied a detailed layout of the apartment and identified the room and the head of the bed in which Hampton would be sleeping. The warrant and the ostensible purpose of the raid were to capture an illegal arms cash, even though O'Neal's inventory of the weapons in the apartment appeared to indicate that all the weapons had been legally acquired. It didn't matter because the weight of the evidence suggests that the real target was Hampton. The raid was rescheduled several times to make sure he would be there. Apparently on instructions from his FBI handler O'Neal had also slipped a sedative into Hampton's drink at a late dinner in the apartment so that he wouldn't wake and would be defenseless. All this information was supplied to the Chicago Police Department's gang intelligence unit, a quasi-secret group under the direction of state's attorney Edward Hanrahan for the conduct of his promised "war on gangs." At 4:30 a.m. on December 4, 1969, fourteen members of the unit arrived at Hampton's apartment armed with a submachine gun, semiautomatic rifles, shotguns, and hand guns. They came without the usual tear gas or loudspeakers, less deadly ways of dealing with a potential confrontation, and issued no surrender warning. Unit members just fired through the front door and broke it down. Over ninety bullets were fired during the raid. Only one bullet came from the Panther side. Mark Clark, sitting with a shotgun by the front door, was shot through the heart and killed instantly by one of the first bullets coming through the front door. The Panther bullet may have come from his gun as he fell to the floor. Hampton never woke up and was killed by two bullets shot at close range to his head. According to two of the Panther survivors from the raid, after hearing the two final shots, they heard a policeman say, "Well, he's sure dead now" (Taylor and Elson 2009, 4). His bloodied body was then dragged out of the bedroom to display as a trophy. Hampton, a voracious reader, left among the books in the bedroom one on how to deliver babies and one on the art of persuasion. His partner, who witnessed the raid, Deborah Johnson, would give birth to their son a few weeks later (Rice 1998, 171–74; Taylor and Elson 2009, 4). He would never have the opportunity to use what he learned from those books in witnessing the birth of his son or in what many of his admirers believed would have been a promising future in law or politics. Both the FBI and the Chicago Police Department were delighted with the "success" of the raid. William O'Neal, who had been paid at least $575 a month over a two-year period, received a $300 bonus from the FBI for his work related to the raid (Rice 1998, 143).

More than five thousand filed past Hampton's coffin at a memorial service on December 9, 1969 (Caputo 1969). Both Jessie Jackson and Ralph Abernathy, director of the SCLC since King's death, delivered eulogies for the twenty-one-year-old Panther leader. Congressional and legal proceedings to uncover the facts related to his death and assign a modicum of responsibility took more than twelve years. Finally, a Seventh Circuit Court of Appeals decision concluded that the FBI and those in the city who planned and carried out the raid had participated in a conspiracy to subvert and eliminate the Black Panther Party and its members and a conspiracy following the raid to cover up the evidence. The Supreme Court refused to overturn the decision, and in February 1983 the federal government, Cook County, and the City of Chicago agreed to settle out of court with the Panther victims for $1.85 million (Taylor and Elson 2009, 6). The defendants never admitted any guilt and dismissed the settlement as just a way to avoid the cost of another trial. For the plaintiffs, it just proved that the police and FBI had gotten away with murder.

The pressure on the Panthers' clinic, part of its more positive image, didn't relent after the killing of Hampton. In January 1970 the city Health Department demanded that the Free Clinic be licensed (*Chicago Tribune* 1970b). Two of the participating physicians, Alfred Klinger and Quentin Young, met with the health commissioner arguing that if the Panthers permitted city licensing, the clinic would be subject to constant harassment (*Chicago Tribune* 1970a). They suggested, as an alternative, getting the participating doctors to incorporate as a group. In February 1970, the Panthers held a rally to protest the threat from the Health Department to close the clinic down. A spokesman for the Young Lords lent its support. "We're here today to show solidarity with the Black Panther party, because we're facing some of the same problems. We feel that when poor black people are attacked, all poor people are being attacked" (*Chicago Daily Defender* 1970). Ronald "Doc" Satchel, the Panther member responsible for organizing the clinic, who was still recovering from five bullet wounds received during the raid of Fred Hampton's apartment, told the demonstrators, "Clinics charging fees and exploiting welfare recipients with assembly line treatment aren't required to have a license. We give residents free treatment and are being harassed" (*Chicago Daily Defender* 1970).

The clinic also had to handle criticism in May 1970 from the president of the Cook County Physicians Association, the local chapter of the NMA, who expressed concern about creating an inadequate dual system of storefront clinics. Satchel pleaded for more understanding. "We have doctors in private practice to refer those patients who need long range care. We have a staff of qualified physicians. . . . We see the medical center, not as a long range solution to the problems of inadequate or no medical care for poor and oppressed people but as an interim thing. We know that it is impossible to care for everyone who needs medical help but we can try and that's exactly what we are doing—trying" (Williams 1970).

By August 1970, the clinic was struggling to get enough physician volunteers. "We are down to about eight doctors out of about 20 in the beginning, and if we don't get more we may have to close down soon" (Nesbit 1970). Satchel said the Panthers were particularly disappointed in the failure of black doctors to participate in the medical program. "Most black doctors are prostituting their skills when they should be given to the people. We urge all black doctors to volunteer at least one evening a week to the community" (qtd. in Nesbit 1970). About 90 percent of the volunteer physicians were white, and this replication of the racial hierarchy of mainstream medicine troubled the Panthers (Schiller 2008, 57). The clinic ceased operating soon afterward. By 1971, as in many other cities, the Illinois chapter of the Panthers ceased to have a physical address and faded from public sight (Caldwell 1971).

The Wounded Street Fighters

The three black medical street fighters with backbone that began the civil right struggle all became casualties as well.

T. R. M. Howard escaped from Mississippi to Chicago under threat of death in 1956 and disappeared from the national civil rights spotlight. He continued to support civil rights causes, including participating in the Committee to End Discrimination in Chicago Medical Institutions. A brilliant but flawed and complicated person, he would not have made a good poster boy for the civil rights movement. In Chicago he embraced an extravagant lifestyle that included a mansion complete with a large room filled with the trophies from his big game hunts in Africa and held lavish parties for Chicago's black elite. Howard supported that lifestyle by becoming the major provider of abortions in Chicago. Abortions did not become legal until the *Roe v. Wade* decision in 1973 (Beito and Beito 2009, 197–228). Howard continued to be a behind-the-scenes financial angel in civil rights causes. He had provided support for the Afro-American Patrolman's League, which courageously bucked the Daly machine and had tried to conduct its own investigation of the death of Fred Hampton. Howard's involvement in abortions had involved criticism from black leaders such Jessie Jackson, whom Howard had given major financial support. A high-quality service, good lawyers, connections, and police bribes kept him out of trouble before the legalization of abortions, but Howard's real troubles were just beginning. His wife, after his fathering of seven illegitimate children and public flaunting of his most recent affair, threw him out of their house and filed for divorce. Lured by Medicaid funding, Howard opened a large, lavish, and dysfunctional clinic, the Freedom Medical Center, in 1972. The overstaffed operation under his inattentive oversight ran up increasing deficits. Faced with growing debt and declining health, Howard died insolvent in May 1976. Friends had to take up a collection to provide him with a gravestone. The death of what some would describe as the father of the modern civil rights movement went unnoticed in the mainstream media.

Sonnie Wellington Hereford III—who integrated the hospital in Huntsville, Alabama, and despite death threats, marched his son to school, defying Governor Wallace, state troopers, and an angry mob, making him the first to integrate a public elementary school in Alabama—did not fare much better. Hereford's patients had always been poor, and he became the major Medicaid provider in Huntsville. Many of Huntsville's white physicians did not accept Medicaid. According to Hereford, he was prosecuted for Medicaid fraud for what on the surface appeared to be relatively minor bookkeeping errors (Hereford and Ellis 2011, 127–49). His medical license was revoked in 1993 for inappropriately prescribing pain medications, but this may have involved just inadequate record keeping. No longer able to practice medicine, Hereford has faced financial difficulties and a painful loss of status in his local community. In general, grudges against activists in the medical profession were slow to heal. In many communities, the black physicians who had waged the hospital desegregation battles were the last black physicians to be provided white hospital privileges.

Reverend Reginald Hawkins, DDS, who had led the civil rights efforts to desegregate public accommodations, schools, and hospitals in Charlotte, North Carolina, remained excluded from the inner circle of the city's leaders. Irrepressible, he had survived the bombing of his home and avoided the bullets of assassins. He died in 2007 at the age of eighty-three, remaining to the end a thorn in the side of Charlotte's Chamber of Commerce. His high point in public recognition came in running in the Democratic primary for governor in 1968. Martin Luther King was scheduled to arrive to help campaign for him the day he was killed in Memphis. His daughter Pauletta was shot and paralyzed, and her three children killed in an execution-style attack in 1973 at a Black Muslim center in Washington, DC, a result of a dispute with the leadership of the black separatist Nation of Islam based in Chicago. It would cast a shadow over the rest of his life (North Carolina History Project 2015).[10]

The lives of all those who had the backbone in the struggle to make "justice flow like water and righteousness like a mighty stream" deserve to be honored. The lives of T. R. M. Howard, Sonnie Hereford, and Reginald Hawkins deserve to be honored as do those of John Chaney, Jean Cowsert, and Fred Hampton.

Death of the Seedbeds

The deaths of two institutions, central to the struggles, deserve to be honored as well—the black hospital and OEHO.

BLACK HOSPITALS

Hospitals are hard to kill. Hospital closings are traumatic events for the communities they serve. A community's hospital provides geographic convenience and a sense of ownership and safety. They are also typically the largest employer in that community. Yet in a period of unprecedented growth and prosperity for historically white hospitals, black ones died. Within two decades of the implementation of Medicare all but four of the more than four hundred twentieth-century historically black hospitals had closed or been converted to other purpose (Wesley 2010). Mound Bayou Hospital (formerly Taborian Hospital), which had helped usher in the post–World War II civil rights struggle with the aid of its first chief of surgery, T. R. M. Howard, closed in 1983. The Reynolds Memorial Hospital in Winston Salem, where Hubert Eaton served his residency had brought the first civil rights case against white hospitals, closed in 1972, leaving vacant a well-equipped modern facility completed just two years earlier. L. Richardson Hospital in Greensboro was the facility used by Dr. George Simkins and local physicians whose suit against the town's white hospitals, Moses Cone and Wesley Long, became Title VI of the Civil Rights Act of 1964 and the foundation from which, with the implementation of Medicare, OEHO was able to mount it initiative to eliminate segregation in all the hospitals in the nation. L. Richardson Hospital, after several attempts to revive it, was sold to a for-profit nursing home chain in 1993. Lincoln Hospital in Durham, where Dr. Charles Watts had served as chief of surgery and where Dr. Paul Cornely—who would later work with W. Montague Cobb at Howard University's medical school on the hospital desegregation battle—did his residency, closed in 1976, when a single regional facility replaced it as well as the historically white hospital in town.

> Durham Regional opened. Lincoln closed down. They tore it down
> and built a new clinic building on the site. Why not maintain
> the old hospital as a landmark? It was erased . . . it had historical
> significance in people's lives. Most things black are torn down. I

suspect people don't want blacks to know their history and some people didn't want to be reminded. . . . Maybe it was just not important to the person making the decision.[11]

Good Samaritan Hospital in Charlotte, North Carolina, the oldest historically black private hospital in the country, and a player in the hospital desegregation campaign launched by Dr. Reginald Hawkins, closed in 1982. The facility was demolished to make way for a stadium for the city's new professional football team, the Charlotte Panthers. A protest demonstration led to the erection of a plaque in the stadium to commemorate the hospital. In 2012, Barack Obama's acceptance speech at the Democratic National Convention was supposed to have been given at that stadium, but the venue had to be changed due to inclement weather.

All the activists responsible for the desegregation that led to the demise of black hospitals felt deeply ambivalent about their passing. Inherent in the situation, Montague Cobb observed, "is the feeling on the part of the Negroes involved that the product of their sweat and toil over the years will be dashed away in the name of progress and that they will find themselves again at the bottom of the ladder where they started" (Cobb 1967, 218–19). Perhaps no truly courageous good deed ever goes unpunished.

OEHO

The high tide of social activism that had been so conducive to the initiation of the OEHO offensive in the spring of 1966 ebbed during the summer. The victories against Jim Crow in the South had sparked increasing frustration with the more intractable de facto discrimination in northern cities, and riots flared up. Casualties mounted in the Vietnam War. Johnson faced an emboldened domestic conservative movement and the beginning of the loss of more liberal allies from opposition to the war. The midterm election in the fall of 1966 resulted in the Republicans gaining three Senate seats, forty-seven House seats, and eight governorships (including Ronald Reagan in California). It signaled an opportunity to thwart Johnson's civil rights initiatives and precipitated OEHO's final death struggle.

The opportunity did not slip by the southern members of Congress, furious with the shell game Gardner had played on them in the temporary shifting of staff to make real Title VI enforcement for hospitals receiving Medicare possible. Centralizing civil rights enforcement in HEW would make it more accountable to Congress. Its budget would be dependent on the House and Senate appropriation committees that shared this responsibility. Instead of the diffusely buried civil rights compliance for public schools, hospitals, and social service programs, they would all be lumped together, located in a single office directly accountable to HEW's secretary and to Congress. The test of wills of the Senate and House appropriations committees with Gardner began shortly after OEHO was set up in February 1966. A March 15, 1966, memo by Assistant Secretary Wilbur Cohen acknowledged in writing the administration's strategy, soon understood by all parties to the HEW appropriations battle.

> At the hearings yesterday before the HEW-Labor Appropriations Subcommittee, Chairman John Fogarty indicated his strong intent to pull out all of the money and positions for civil rights enforcement in separate places where they are now and lump them in one appropriation. . . . Whatever merits this proposal might have it has one serious defect: *It will highlight the substantial number of positions involved in civil rights enforcement and serve as a basis for cutting the appropriations and the number of positions.* (Cohen 1966, italics added)

For a critical year, Gardner and HEW had defied the will of Congress. On May 4, 1966, Representative John Fogarty (D, RI), chairman of the House appropriations subcommittee, reported that HEW's spending for civil rights activities was "budgeted in a great many different places in the department. The committee deleted these every place they occurred and has consolidated the funds in the office of the secretary. The committee believes that this will provide a much more efficient and effective program. . . . I recognize that a period of transition and experimentation will be necessary. A major part of the department's civil rights effort must be carried out through the regional offices, so the secretary should have some discretion and flexibility in allocating civil rights personnel to regional offices" (qtd. in Steif 1967, 2–3). At the end of the summer of 1966 most of those on temporary assignment to OEHO had drifted back to their home agencies. Gardner stalled, agreeing that the centralization would be studied, gaining the critical time necessary for carrying out the Medicare Title VI hospital compliance initiative. In the spring of 1967, however, the demand for centralization was renewed and with it the threat that the entire HEW appropriation would be held up if it was not implemented. The new chairman of the HEW appropriations subcommittee, Representative Daniel Flood (D, PA) held hearings and got lots of testimony from southern congressmen about "misenforcement" of the Civil Rights Act. Flood reported to Gardner that "members of the subcommittee are seriously concerned with certain contentions made by outside witnesses about the department's approach to enforcement . . . and are particularly disturbed that the department has not been fully responsive to the committee report last year calling for complete centralization of civil rights enforcement staff," and when the secretary provided his plans, they would "assist the subcommittee in its consideration of the 1968 budget" (qtd. in Steif 1967, 4). The southerners wanted an end to targeting Jim Crow segregated schools in the South while not treating de facto segregation in northern cities similarly, and they wanted civil rights enforcement centralized. The backlash had begun, and if HEW failed to comply they could expect big cuts in funds. On May 10, 1967, Gardner announced the reorganization at a press conference. It was announced formally in the *Federal Register* on October 9, 1967. The transfer of staff and functions began late in the summer of 1967 and would be completed in the winter of 1968. The intent of this centralization, as far as any involved in the Title VI hospital certification process were concerned, had nothing to do with efficiency and improved coordination. Its intent was Congress's desire to control the effort and clip its wings.

Robert Nash, director of OEHO, refused reassignment to the centralized office, and many others who had been part of the core of OEHO either refused reassignment to the centralized office or left soon after the centralization. Bobby Childers, who had been director of the Charlottesville regional office OEHO operation, chose to leave rather than remain in the centralized Office for Civil Rights. "I got ticked off and left with the change in administration. The Republicans came in and wouldn't let you do anything. They went about the school desegregation totally wrong. They should have made the states enforce Title VI, instead they by passed the states."[12] Marilyn Rose, who had served as counsel to Robert Nash, left HEW in March 1968. "At this point the health civil rights program was on the skids. The referral practices issue was dead after the Mobile cave-in and the Department also virtually abandoned any real attempt to desegregate the nursing home industry" (Rose 1997, 13–14). Gardner wrote his letter of resignation in January 1968 and delivered it in person to President Johnson. The Vietnam War, the urban riots, and the civil rights backlash were part of the course of events that led to this decision. He told Johnson that he had concluded that he should not run for a second term. Libassi joined him in resigning, and Wilbur Cohen became HEW secretary for the remainder of Johnson's term. Johnson himself soon decided not to run for a second term. The Tet Offensive in Vietnam and rising opposition to the war at home, along with Martin Luther King's assassination and the subsequent riots in Washington, DC, Chicago, and elsewhere, crowded out any public or official attention to health care priorities.

The short, happy life of the Office of Equal Health Opportunity was over. It had served as the high point in the career of many civil servants and as a high point in federal efforts to end racial segregation. It had been a liberating experience that neither the individuals nor the federal bureaucracy would ever capture again. Almost all the staffing in the new office focused on the problems of school desegregation which, through the efforts of southern legislators, now required "equal treatment" with northern de facto segregation. Under Wilbur Cohen, who had assumed the position of secretary for the remainder of Johnson's term, civil rights compliance ceased to be a pervasive focus of HEW. OEHO had reflected the passion and spirit of the civil rights movement. As that movement fragmented, it seemed almost inevitable that OEHO would reflect that disintegration and just fade away.

The newly created centralized Office for Civil Rights, with the Nixon election in November 1968, faced two incompatible responsibilities on a collision course: keep peace on the Hill (that is, with Congress) and enforce the civil rights law. Nixon and White House staff, as a part of a "southern strategy" (Wallace had carried Alabama, Arkansas, Georgia, Louisiana, and Mississippi, and Nixon won the election with only 43.4 percent to Humphrey's 42.7 percent of the popular vote), had apparently made promises to southern legislatures to back off on aggressive enforcement. Leon Panetta, the new director of the Office for Civil Rights, proceeded with trying to enforce the law while Senator Strom Thurmond (R, SC) demanded that the White House keep its promises. One version of what happened next, differing only slightly in details from Panetta's own recollections, comes from a former OEHO staff member transferred to OCR (Panetta and Gill 1971, see 350–67).

> One day I went down to mail a letter. As I went to the corner to mail it, this guy tosses a bundle of newspapers off the delivery truck. The wire was still on them but I noticed the headline: "Panetta Resigns." . . . When I go back into the office Panetta's Secretary tells me, "He's in a meeting, you can't go in." I said, "I think he needs to see this," I go in and flash the headline at him. "Jesus! What the hell is this?" he says. Anyway, it seems that that a Senator had announced on the Senate Floor that Panetta had resigned and that's where the headline came from. Leon called Secretary Finch to find out what was going on and the Secretary had a call from the White House asking him what he knew about it. There had been no resignation and the White House hadn't asked for one.[13]

Soon afterward, asked at a press conference, Nixon's press secretary, Ron Ziegler, confirmed that "Panetta had submitted his resignation and it had been accepted." The Nixon White House had offered Panetta as a sacrificial lamb to placate the southern legislators. Panetta then wrote a resignation letter. A petition signed by many HEW civil servants protested these events (Panetta and Gill 1971). Finch was relieved of his duties as secretary a few weeks later. Perhaps chastened by the uproar, Nixon's OCR subsequently achieved some progress in desegregating southern school districts.

During the Carter reorganization in 1979 civil rights efforts in education and health were once again divided, but the health component got only a small fraction of the staff (staffing was roughly divided on the basis of complaints, and parents of school children are much more likely to complain than patients).[14] Little of the original spirit of OEHO survived these reorganizations, and little of the civil rights movement pressures that had forced such significant changes remained.

On my own visit to OCR in 2014, Panetta's account of his brief tenure as OCR director, *Bring Us Together: The Nixon Team and the Civil Rights Retreat*, was prominently displayed on the coffee table in the office of Leon Rodriquez, then OCR director. "I put it there as a reminder that one should never be afraid of losing one's job for enforcing the law," he said.[15] Sparks from the old flame persist.[16]

Morning in America?

As the civil rights tide ebbed, faced with the almost intractable difficulties of addressing the invisible color lines of de facto segregation, opposition became more sophisticated in framing the debate in a coded language that never mentioned race, segregation, or discrimination. The total war launched by the Mississippi Sovereignty Commission and the FBI COINTELPRO became privatized into well-funded think tanks and political action committees unrestrained by budgets or public accountability. The erasing of history began.

Ronald Reagan made his first speech after being nominated as the Republican Party's candidate for president on August 3, 1980, at the Neshoba County Fairground near Philadelphia, Mississippi, a few miles from where the bodies of James Chaney, Michael Schwerner, and Andrew Goodman had been found on August 4, 1964, sixteen years earlier. Amid lighthearted jokes about Carter and self-deprecating remarks about himself, the impromptu speech included these lines: "I still believe the answer to any problem lies with the people. I believe in states' rights and I believe in people doing as much as they can for themselves at the community level and at the private level. I believe we have distorted the balance of our government today by giving powers that were never intended to be given in the Constitution to that federal establishment" (Reagan 1980). Reagan went on to promise to "restore to states and local governments the power that properly belongs to them" (Reagan 1980).

The speech finalized the transformation of Dixiecrats to Republicans. Everyone understood what it meant, but many were never convinced that Reagan really meant it. Just like John Gardner, Reagan, no matter what his intent, had the magic of couching everything in a universal feel-good language. In the early years after World War II, Reagan had even shared membership in the pro–civil rights American Veteran's Committee with many who would become key civil rights activists in the 1960s.

For those who still embrace the dream of the civil rights movement, those who have seen its glory, the struggle isn't over. Perhaps they should take their cues from both Gardner and Reagan. Maybe it can still be morning in America.

6

Seen the Glory

> Well, I don't know what will happen now. We've got
> some difficult days ahead. . . . But I want you to know
> tonight, that we, as a people, will get to the Promised
> Land. And I'm happy, tonight. I'm not worried
> about anything. I'm not fearing any man. Mine eyes
> have seen the glory of the coming of the Lord.
> —Martin Luther King, Memphis, April 3, 1968 (King 1968)

Buried beneath all the events that captured the headlines and television news footage, the civil rights movement quietly attended to the
birth of Medicare. The movement changed health care more than any
other aspect of American life. It transformed the nation's most racially
and economically segregated institutions into its most integrated. The
movement tore down most of the walls of a starkly separate and unequal system. The exhilaration of these accomplishments sent shock
waves through the rest of society. It was, perhaps, the civil rights movement's most glorious gift. This final chapter describes that gift and the
promise it still offers.

Rising Again

What happened in health care, of course, can't be separated from the
larger civil rights story. That story didn't end with the "civil rights era,"
despite all its casualties, and its rising again has been its true glory.
Resilience, persistence, and ingenuity have helped forged new paths
toward that "Promised Land." The Chicago Freedom Movement's premature obituary marking the end of the civil rights era, for example,
needs updating.

In 1966, the Chicago Freedom Movement (CFM) came to the same conclusion that academic research and those in public policy would come to much later: residential segregation was a root cause of unequal opportunity. Segregation and disparities in hospital care, for example, persist today not primarily because of discrimination by individual hospitals or their medical staffs but because of the racial and economic segregation of the neighborhoods in which they are located. Place shapes the resources a hospital has and the health problems it faces. For example, the discharged patients from a hospital in a neighborhood with a high poverty rate are less likely to have access to good primary and home care and, as a consequence, are more likely to be readmitted to that hospital. Residential segregation similarly shapes educational and employment opportunities. Just as with hospital desegregation efforts with the implementation of Medicare, only a structural, system-wide solution can address the problem.

In conjunction with the CFMs protest marches in 1966, a lawsuit was filed, *Dorothy Gautreaux v. Chicago Housing Authority*, by Chicago Housing Authority (CHA) residents with the assistance of American Civil Liberties Union lawyers (see Polikoff 2006). The suit alleged that the CHA's use of federal Housing and Urban Development (HUD) funds violated Title VI. Indeed, between 1954 and 1967, CHA had constructed more than 10,300 public housing units with only sixty-three built outside poor, racially segregated areas. A matching suit brought against HUD for permitting the use of federal funds in this manner resulted in a Supreme Court decision ten years later (Hills v. Gautreaux 425 US 284). The court ordered HUD to provide scattered-site housing for CHA residents living in impoverished, racially segregated neighborhoods in predominantly white and more affluent neighborhoods *throughout the entire Chicago metropolitan area*. Despite many difficulties, by the end of 1998 the Gautreaux program had succeeded in relocating seventy-two hundred families from segregated, impoverished neighborhoods into private rental housing (section 8) in predominantly white, higher-income areas throughout Chicago and its suburbs. The implementation, just as Medicare's Title VI enforcement, was a quiet, low-profile effort. Only one or two units were acquired in any neighborhood to avoid white flight and the overwhelming of local services. Just as Medicare's hospital desegregation effort had worked mostly with private sector hospitals, the Gautreaux project circumvented local public officials and just arranged for the rental of private housing. Local governments could have blocked the construction of public housing units, but the Gautreaux project flew under the radar. The program was a popular one among potentially eligible families and won bipartisan presidential support from Carter, Reagan, and Bush, and eventually fifty programs modeled after it were in place across the country.

Those promising results, combined with the riots in South Central Los Angeles in 1992, produced section 154 of the Housing and Community Development Act of 1992. It launched a more rigorous and ambitious HUD experiment, Moving to Opportunity. Moving to Opportunity essentially replicated the Gautreaux model, randomly assigning households to a "control" and a "treatment" group in five cities (Baltimore, Boston, Chicago, Los Angeles, and New York).

Moving to Opportunity produced improvements in the health, educational attainments, and employment for families in the treatment group. There were, for example, modest but potentially important reductions in the prevalence of obesity and diabetes in those participating in the relocation as opposed to the controls (Ludwig et al. 2011). The most recent evaluation of this effort indicates that it resulted in significant improvements in college attendance rates and earnings of children who were below the age of thirteen when they moved. To quote the researchers, "The findings imply that offering families with young children living in high-poverty housing projects vouchers to move to lower poverty neighborhoods may reduce the intergeneration persistence of poverty and ultimately generate positive returns for taxpayers" (Chetty, Hendren, and Katz 2015, 1). Simultaneous with the release of these findings the US Department of Housing and Urban Development (HUD) issued new rules, reminiscent of the Title VI guidelines issued to hospitals fifty years ago, requiring cities to set goals for reducing segregation in housing or face the potential withholding of HUD funding for their failure to meet them (Trott 2015). Integration, being all in it together, works not just for hospitals but in addressing one of the fundamental root causes of disparities in general, residential segregation. In the long run, the dismantling of urban ghettoes not only is feasible but could save taxpayers money.

Even the seeming violent demise of the Chicago Black Panthers failed in blocking its more resilient and generous legacy. Some of the Panther Free Clinics in city ghettos morphed into Federally Qualified Neighborhood Health Centers (Schiller 2008). The Breakfast for Children Program of the Panthers morphed into the School Breakfast Program, permanently authorized by Congress in 1975, which now provides breakfast for sixteen million low-income children. The Panthers' campaign to address sickle cell anemia was enacted into law by Richard Nixon in the National Sickle Cell Anemia Control Act of 1972. It, combined with the Medicare and Medicaid programs, continues to provide substantial federal funding to screen, assist in the care for victims of this ailment, and explore better treatment options. The Panthers, transformed into mainstream political organizers, defeated the reelection of state's attorney Edward Harahan, who was responsible for the raid that cost Fred Hampton's life and for the subsequent cover-up. The "Panthers' coalition" with Hispanics elected Chicago's first black mayor, Harold Washington, in 1983. Bobby Rush, who replaced Hampton as chairman of the Illinois Panthers after his death, was elected to Congress in 1991 from the First Congressional District of Illinois and continues to serve as its congressman. In 2000 Barack Obama, then a state senator and political neophyte, challenged Rush for his seat in the Democratic primary. Rush crushed him. Still concerned about access and health disparities, Congressman Rush in a 2015 interview noted, "There are still too many sick people, people who are chronically ill, people who have serious, serious health issues and they have inadequate access to health care. . . . Here we are some fifty plus years later, and we still have a very, very serious problem in terms of access."[1] Rush is also a part of the Panther and Fred Hampton legacy.

The Glory

Indeed, the world of health care now bears little resemblance to the one that existed in the formative years described in the first chapter. That world took color lines for granted, enforced either by Jim Crow laws or by the invisible barriers of residential segregation and medical practice patterns. It took for granted the differences in access to care between the more affluent and the poor. It restricted the opportunities of black medical professionals. All of this was "just the way things were."[2]

What happened changed how care was allocated and narrowed the disparities in care that blacks and low-income persons received. It produced system-wide changes that make all the efforts at reform and quality improvement in health care since then insignificant by comparison.

Not only did all the visible symbols of Jim Crow disappear, but in a decade the entire structure of institutional care changed. All but four or five of the more than four hundred black hospitals that had existed in the twentieth century either closed or were converted to other purposes (Wesley 2010). Most of the public hospitals that had exclusively served the indigent also either closed or were converted to facilities that also served the economic mainstream. The change happened so quickly that many did not believe it had really happened at all. New facilities replaced the aging black ones at the end of the 1960s, only to be abandoned by their former patients and physicians, who were now welcomed at the formerly racially or economically segregated white institutions.

Within facilities, not only did the racial separations disappear immediately, but, more gradually, the economic segregation of patients decreased as well. The separation of private and public inpatient accommodations, with few exceptions, no longer exist. The twenty-bed open charity wards in hospitals disappeared, replaced by private and semiprivate rooms shared equally by all income and racial groups. The common hospital practice of three sets of dishes, silverware, furniture, and menus to mark a patient's position in the social hierarchy also disappeared. The wooden benches and block scheduling of indigent clinics have also mostly disappeared. Clinic accommodations for indigent patients are now, for the most part, indistinguishable from those in private office practices. The racially separate waiting rooms in private physician practices, responding to the lead of the hospitals and the new economic power of black Medicare beneficiaries, also disappeared soon after the color barriers came down in hospitals, even in the most politically conservative practices in the Deep South.

Profound changes also took place in access to care. Within a decade the "iron law" that had distributed use of services by race and income, inversely related to actual need for more than half a century during the formative years of modern medicine, was turned on its head (Smith 1999, 200–210). In the Medicare program, expenditures per nonwhite beneficiary gradually increased to the point where they exceeded hospital expenditures per white beneficiary (Smith 1999, 206). Age-adjusted hospital discharges and days of care for blacks and for low-income persons both now substantially exceed those for whites and high-income persons (Smith 1999, 203). Age-adjusted black physician contacts per year, which were only 77 percent of white contacts, rose to 96 percent of whites by 1980; and low-income contacts, which were only 75 percent of high-income contacts in 1964 rose to 120 percent of high-income contacts per year by 1980 (Smith 1999, 202). For the first time in the history of medicine in the United States, patterns of use actually began to reflect patterns of need. The moral duty of hospitals and physicians to care for the sick, which had been little more than lip service, began for the first time to be reflected in actual statistical patterns of use.

The changes also began to narrow the differences in the health of racial and economic groups for the first time. Racial and economic differences in rates of premature death (death before sixty-five) and infant mortality (deaths before one year of age) shrank in the United States between 1964 and 1980 (Krieger et al. 2008). Racial disparities in death rates were more directly related to improvement in access as a result of the desegregation of hospitals in the South (infant mortality and deaths due to motor vehicle accidents also declined markedly during this same period; Almond, Chay, and Greenstone 2008; Zheng and Zhou 2009). While since the 1980s such "differences" have budged little, they have at least been cast in a different light, as "disparities," an inequity that is unjust and that providers of care have a moral and legal obligation to do whatever they can to eliminate. That small shift in language represented a profound cultural shift.

As a result, significant changes have occurred in the three pillars of the American health care system, erected during its formative years: (1) volunteerisms, (2) duty to neglect, and (3) exploitation of the vulnerable have been shaken at their foundations.

Volunteerism is no longer voluntary. Volunteerism implied private freedom not public responsibility. Through its role as a recipient of federal funding health care's voluntary sector has become a quasi-public one. Indeed, voluntary hospitals, according to the *Simkins* decision, which paved the way for their desegregation, were defined as "an arm of the state." The "voluntary" Blue Cross plans became third-party administrators of Medicare and some Medicaid plans, relying on them for a substantial portion of their revenues. Hospitals, originally defined as private charities, soon after the passage of Medicare lost their private charitable immunity from malpractice. Even the epitome of the private, voluntary, professional approach for assuring hospital standards, the Joint Commission for Accreditation of Healthcare Organizations (JCAHO), became a partner of Medicare in certifying hospitals for Medicare payments. The tax exempt status of private voluntary hospitals as charities has also been increasingly challenged by both local and federal governments for those institutions that stray too far from their public responsibilities. The Affordable Care Act, in addition, requires all nonprofit hospitals, in planning their services, to do triennial community needs assessments or face penalties.

Duty to neglect has become neglect of duty. The chasm between need and use of care has closed. The Emergency Medical Treatment and Active Labor Act (EMTALA) requires hospitals to provide emergency treatment and prevents the dumping of patients lacking citizenship, legal status, or the ability to pay.[3] In addition, hospital systems, in response to their need to get Medicare and Medicaid revenues from admissions, are increasingly imposing as a condition for medical staff privileges a willingness to accept such payments.[4]

Exploitation of the vulnerable doesn't work for those that are now paying patients with choices. Research and teaching hospitals have faced increasing competition for what they had previously taken for granted as a necessary but unwelcomed obligation. That previously unwelcomed obligation became a critical resource for their fiscal, research, and educational survival. As a result, most research and teaching hospitals have made continuous renovations and service improvements to attract and keep their medically indigent patient population. The charity wards, wooden bench, block-scheduled clinics have all disappeared. The amenities of clinics in most cities now match or exceed those of private office practices. In addition, the human subject controls put in place as a result of the Tuskegee syphilis experiment, which became a scandal only after the implementation of Medicare and Medicaid, have helped, as have the resulting tighter controls over federal research funding.

The Shock Waves

The success in enforcing Title VI with the implementation of Medicare marked a watershed for the federal government. It transformed it from the passive, compliant partner supplying funds for private entities and local governments into a powerful force for equal treatment. The first attempt by the federal government to impose equal opportunity requirements on an entire private sector receiving federal funds came with the implementation of the Medicare program. That principle, embodied in Title VI of the Civil Rights Act of 1964, had been the product of a bitter political and legal battle that had taken more than a decade to enact. Its success in ending the racial segregation of hospitals opened a floodgate of change. Similar requirements soon changed the landscape of higher education. Single-sex colleges and universities almost disappeared in the next decade. Professional schools of medicine, law, and business, previously exclusive male bastions, soon served student bodies that are about half female. Others discriminated against by disability or sexual orientation soon benefited from requirements for equal opportunity in organizations receiving federal funding.

The most profound shock wave, however, went unnoticed at the time. It involved the federal government's applying to itself the same rules it was applying to those it was funding. In October 1965, just two months after signing the Medicare legislation, President Lyndon Johnson signed the Immigration and Naturalization Act of 1965, with the Statue of Liberty in the background. While Liberty had held up her light by the golden door, she had permitted only white, predominantly northern European immigrants through it. The new law eliminated these racial, ethnic, and geographic restrictions.

The Immigration and Naturalization Act of 1965 thus launched the second "Great Migration." The first Great Migration, begun some fifty years earlier, relocated millions of blacks seeking a better life from the Deep South to northern cities. The second, over the next fifty years, produced perhaps an even more profound shift. While the number of foreign-born Europeans in the nation would decline, the total foreign-born would increase fourfold. The number of Asians would increase twenty-two-fold to more than eleven million. The number of Latin American foreign-born would increase twenty-three-fold to twenty-two million. The number of individuals born in Africa residing in the United States increased forty-five-fold to 1.6 million (US Bureau of the Census 1960, 2010).

Demographics became destiny, despite the initial political requisites—money and the vote. The first Great Migration delivered the presidential election victory of John F. Kennedy in 1960, which began the federal civil rights offensive. The second Great Migration delivered the presidential election victories of Barack Obama in 2008 and more decisively in 2012.

In assuring access to health care, the second migration stood on the shoulders of the first. The Supreme Court concluded in *Lau v. Nichols* (1973) that the prohibition in Title VI against discrimination on the basis of "national origin" was a proxy for language and that recipients of federal funding could be found liable for discrimination for failing to provide access to language services. With little of the hospital resistance that blacks experienced earlier, hospitals embraced the jointly agreed-on Culturally and Linguistically Appropriate Services (CLAS) Standards for handling the language and cultural problems this new wave of immigrants face in receiving care. It was a rational response that was lacking in the original struggle to racially desegregate hospitals. No hospital, after all, wants to turn away any paying customers nor expose themselves to the malpractice risks of not being able to communicate with its patients. Both migrations were the consequence of the decisions of powerless, disenfranchised individuals seeking a better life. Yet collectively they transformed the nation's cultural, social, and political life. One can't help but "see the glory" in such a transformation.

Quieting Trouble

> The system basically stays the same. It
> only gives enough to quiet trouble.
> —Reverend Fred Shuttlesworth (qtd. in Galloway 1999, B1)[5]

Such a brief convulsive period, of course, left many things unchanged, and existing institutions blunted the changes that did take place. Indeed, if slavery was a peculiar institution of the antebellum South, the health care system of the United States as it exists today is a similarly peculiar accommodation between its pre–civil rights era formative years and the demands of the civil rights revolution.

Jim Crow practices didn't really segregate the races in the way that is often assumed today. Indeed, then just as now, the South was more racially integrated than the North. Today, largely reflecting the lower degree of residential segregation in most southern cities, both hospitals and nursing homes in the South have the lowest degree of segregation of any region in the country (Smith 1998; Smith et al. 2007). What Jim Crow practices did do was impose rules on what blacks could and couldn't do in occupying the same space as whites. Harry Golden, Charlotte, North Carolina, journalist, activist and close friend of Carl Sandburg, famously made much fun of these rules in the 1950s (Golden 1958). For example, blacks in many segregated hospitals were perfectly free to wait in integrated lines at the hospital pharmacy for prescriptions. They just couldn't sit next to each other in a waiting area and couldn't occupy a bed in the same room next to a white person.

Both sitting and lying down next to each other implied a degree of interracial equality and intimacy that was unacceptable. Thus, Golden observed, "vertical integration" was perfectly acceptable. With this insight, Golden proposed that the problem of school desegregation in the South could be easily solved—all you had to do was to remove all the chairs and let the students remain standing. "They're not learning to read sitting down," Golden observed, "maybe standing up will help" (Golden 1967, 220).

Vertical integration but horizontal segregation in terms of health care was, unfortunately, more than just a tongue-in-cheek joke. It seems to have become the guide for how health care should be reorganized in the United States after the civil rights era. Hospitals proceeded to "quiet trouble" in accommodating to the Title VI prohibition against discrimination in room assignments in two ways.

First, whenever possible, hospital rooms were converted to private, single-bed ones that made the problem of racial matching by room disappear. Much of the boom in new construction of hospitals, ironically, financed by Hill-Burton grants and Medicare capital cost payments, facilitated this transformation. In Mobile, Alabama, site of the last bitter OEHO battle over hospital desegregation, all the hospitals converted to single-occupancy rooms. Providence Hospital, ironically the one that paved the way in desegregating, relocated, following a pattern replicated by hospital relocations in many northern cities, to a more predominantly affluent and white part of Mobile. In Raleigh-Durham, North Carolina, the new "integrated" regional hospital that merged the older black and white hospitals serving the city provided private, single-bed accommodations for its patients. Indeed, the same solution was adopted in many facilities in urban areas in the North, whose service areas overlapped white and black segregated residential areas.

Second, in conjunction with this and in the event that single-bed accommodations were not possible, hospitals could just reduce the length of stay. As noted in Chapter 3, both the University of North Carolina and the University of Mississippi Medical Centers adopted this approach, first integrating their intensive care units, where most of the patients were comatose and not capable of protesting. Indeed, with the shift in acuity of patients cared for, acute care hospitals as a whole have almost been transformed into intensive care units. New forms of payment by Medicare and other hospital insurers provided additional incentives for reducing length of stay in the 1980s. The average length of stay dropped more than 30 percent, the number of hospital days per one thousand population in the United States dropped more than 40 percent, and the number of acute community hospital beds dropped to 2.6 beds per one thousand in 2011. The beds per one thousand population in the United States is now less than 60 percent of what it was in 1980 (National Center for Health Statistics 2014, 299, 314, 322). (The decline in occupancy also helped to facilitate the conversion of semi-private rooms into private ones.) As a result, the United States now has the lowest number of beds per one thousand population and the lowest length of stay of any affluent country in the world. Indeed, the number of hospital beds per one thousand population in the United States is now less than half the average of high-income Organization for Economic and Cooperative Development (OECD) countries ("Countries Compared by Health" 2015). The most common explanation for the reduction in length of stay in the United States is that "it saves money." That explanation just doesn't hold up. Why then, would hospital costs per capita in the United States be twice that in any other developed country despite the smaller supply of hospital beds and fewer days of hospital care?

Even Harry Golden's joke about solving the school desegregation problem by removing the chairs reflected some of the actual adjustments hospitals made in desegregating their facilities. For example, Mobile General Hospital, the public facility that was a participant in the last bitter struggle by OEHO to enforce both the letter and the spirit of the Title VI requirements on hospitals, actually made use of Golden's proposal. Concerned with avoiding the possibility of racial confrontations in its main lobby after integration, all the seating was removed. In its place, medical staff members were asked to scour the attics for the artifacts of their physician ancestors that could be used to fill display cases in the lobby. The cases displayed the surgical instruments used by physician ancestors who had served in the Confederate Army during the Civil War.[6] It had to have been a source of amusement among the exhibit's suppliers, a grand act of defiance against the Yankee invaders. Almost forty years later, after an appraisal suggested that this priceless collection should be better protected against theft, a fund-raising effort relocated the collection to a more secure home for the exhibits in a "medical museum." By then almost no institutional memory existed about why the collection had been located in the lobby in the first place. It just no longer seemed right for the hospital's patients to be greeted on their arrival with the hardly comforting sight of rusty instruments used in amputating limbs. Some seating arrangements were finally returned to the lobby.

Unfortunately, the net effect of the shift in patterns of hospital use in the United States was to backslide, adding to the challenges health care's most vulnerable populations face in getting care and, to a certain extent, resegregating it. Ambulatory care and home care resources are much more a function of the relative wealth or poverty of the neighborhoods patients reside in. Wealthy neighborhoods have more resources than poor ones. In most urban areas those neighborhoods are segregated by race and income, and so are the services. Readmission rates to hospitals are in part a function of the adequacy of the resources available in different communities to care for discharged patients. Hospitals that serve blacks and predominately lower-income neighborhoods have higher readmission rates (Joynt, Oray, and Jha 2011). Incentives to hospitals for low readmission rates tend to punish hospitals that serve low-income and minority communities rather than reward effectiveness. Many hospitals now provide additional outreach services to help forestall readmissions since they now face Medicare financial penalties (Center for Medicare and Medicaid Services 2015). Wouldn't it be less costly for the system as a whole just to extend lengths of stays?

The Johnson administration and Secretary Gardner's HEW, unfortunately, sought to "quiet trouble" as well. Their approach focused just on the "low-hanging fruit"—the nation's acute community hospitals. For these hospitals, complying with Title VI meant the difference between getting the Medicare funding necessary for profitable growth and almost inevitable insolvency. It was also impossible for them to fake compliance. The guidelines were clear, and their own patients, employees, and even some medical staff would blow the whistle if they attempted to circumvent them. HEW chose, however, to exempt private practice physicians from Title VI. The ostensible reason for doing so was that the Civil Rights Act of 1964 Title VI exempted federal "contracts of insurance or guaranties." It is not clear whether that exclusion legally really extended to Part B of Medicare. It did, however, quiet a lot of trouble. Trying to enforce Title VI in some 250,000 independent private medical practices that would receive Medicare payments under Part B would have been a nightmare. In the pre-electronic billing and medical record world of private practice in 1966, there would have been no way to audit compliance. No one, certainly not the physicians, wanted to be party to a policing process that prescribed who physicians agreed to accept as a patient or how they treated them. Any attempt to enforce Title VI in Part B payments to physicians would have turned the rumors of a threatened boycott after the passage of Medicare in July 1965 into a reality.

The problem, of course, as the case of the Mobile Infirmary illustrated, is that desegregating hospitals would be a hollow gesture in the face of an independent and civil rights–recalcitrant medical staff. The saving grace, however, as it turned out, was that, except for a few old-guard outliers, physicians followed the lead of the hospitals where they had privileges. For most, transparently racially discriminatory behavior was professionally abhorrent. In addition, Medicare Part B usual and customary fee schedules were generous, and it made no sense as a rational business model for a practice to accept or treat black Medicare beneficiaries any differently than white ones. Medicare made no racial distinctions in the generosity of these payments.

Today most physicians are contractually tied to a variety of health plans and many to hospital-health systems, which are capable of imposing any kind of electronic monitoring of practices that makes sense in assuring access, quality, and cost effectiveness. Yet some racial and economic disparities, particularly in referrals for some forms of specialty care, persist. Perhaps trouble has been quieted for too long.

Quieting Title VI trouble, however, shaped a profound transformation of medical care facilities far beyond the boundaries of community hospitals. The first victim of the November 1966 midterm election backlash was the Title VI compliance program for nursing homes. Forms similar to the ones sent to hospitals in March of 1966 had been sent out to all the nation's nursing homes, scheduled to begin participation in the Medicare program six months after the hospitals, in January 1967.

> We had all worked very hard from eight o'clock in the morning to eight or nine in the evening. We had hoped to develop some kind of formula from the forms, to follow-up on nursing homes, as we had done with the hospitals. Nevertheless, President Johnson had decided during the first part of 1967 that he was not going to require anything. All he was going to do is require a good faith effort. The nursing homes had to advertise in the local newspaper classified section that they were nondiscriminatory. . . . They

couldn't use very small print but nothing large bold print was required. I didn't like that, but I understood why, because nursing homes are different from hospitals. . . . It is as much a social kind of environment as a medical one. There were also nursing home associations and politicians from the South who ran a lot of committees then, who said if you don't do that, you're going to lose votes. I don't know if I had been in President Johnson's shoes then that I would have done differently. Nevertheless, I was disappointed.[7]

Nursing home segregation and discrimination never became a civil rights issue. Nobody wanted to go to a nursing home in the first place. For blacks, the history of the use of county farms and workhouses in the South to discipline the black plantation labor force after the Civil War blurred into their transformation into nursing homes, adding to their aversion. It was hard to portray discrimination in access to such facilities as a burning civil rights issue. In addition, unlike hospital staff privileges, which were critical for the livelihood of a physician, seeing patients in a nursing home became regarded as an under-reimbursed burden. Black physicians who had pressed for the desegregation of hospital medical staffs had little interest in pressing for similar "privileges" in nursing homes. Medicare also had much less financial leverage over nursing homes. It accounted for less than 10 percent of the income of homes, the rest flowing from the out-of-pocket payments of patients and from state-operated Medicaid programs for the medically indigent. As a result, nursing homes continue to operate as a more tiered and segregated system (Smith et al. 2007; Smith et al. 2008; Mor et al. 2004).

Institutions, no matter what their purported purpose, are not insulated silos. The individuals using general hospitals, nursing homes, mental hospitals, and prisons migrate between these facilities depending on the advantages they offer to those controlling the flow of admissions and discharges in either shifting costs or quieting trouble. As indicated in Figure 1, a massive relocation of people among these institutions took place in the wake of the civil rights era and the implementation of the Medicare and Medicaid programs.

The rapid expansion of stand-alone nursing homes produced a three-and-a half-fold increase in nursing home use. Nursing home bed capacity more than doubled between 1963 and 1973, to more 1.175 million beds, exceeding the bed capacity of acute care hospitals (National Center for Health Statistics 1975). Many acute care hospitals with a complement of nursing home beds in an adjoining wing closed them to pursue the financial incentives Medicare offered for acute care and, possibly perhaps, to quiet possible trouble that Title VI requirements might pose for nursing homes operated by an acute care hospital. Much of the new capacity of the nursing home sector was filled by elderly residents from state psychiatric hospitals. While many had ended up in state mental hospitals as a way to shift the cost of their care from local hospitals and counties to state government, many were now shifted to the newly emerging private nursing home sector to shift some of the cost of their care to the federal government. Medicare and Medicaid do not pay for non-acute care in hospitals for the mentally ill.[8] The federal government chose not to assume the added burden of what had historically been a state responsibility. For nursing home care, however, whatever the state Medicaid program paid for such care, the federal government would at least match. For poorer states the federal share was much higher. For example, in Alabama each dollar would be matched with $2.32 in federal dollars, and for Mississippi every dollar the state spent would be matched with $2.87 (Kaiser Family Foundation 2015a). No state official looking at such numbers had any problem figuring how to make the most out of their budgets for chronic care. For states that had historically operated separate black mental hospitals, such as Alabama, Georgia, Mississippi, and Virginia, it provided an added incentive to shift patients to either ambulatory or nursing home care, both of which were reimbursable under Medicaid. The state could then shift much of the cost for the care of the medically indigent onto the federal government. As a result, state mental hospital institutionalization rates declined to less than 5 percent of their rates fifty years ago (Sisti, Segal, and Emanuel 2015). Most of the state hospitals closed. Their former residents have, for the most part, not been "deinstitutionalized." They have just been, as Figure 1 suggests, "reinstitutionalized" into the expanded capacity of nursing homes and prisons.

The most dramatic growth in institutionalization came in the 1980s with a fourfold increase in incarceration rates. Prisons are now the major institutional provider of services for the mentally ill. The United States has the highest incarceration rates in the world, and black males have incarceration rates six times those of white males. Unlike the other shifts in institutional rates there is no budgetary benefit to state and local governments for such a shift. The federal government's Medicare and Medicaid programs provide no matching funds to prisons or prisoners. It is acknowledged by most thoughtful observers as the most costly and destructive way to quiet trouble, a way that has been quite appropriately labeled the "New Jim Crow" (Alexander 2012). The beginning of a decline in incarceration rates perhaps reflects a more hopeful, or at least fiscally rational, emerging bipartisan consensus.

While Figure 1 summarizes the statistical trends, it doesn't convey the sad and sometimes brutal stories that underlie them. The recent decline in nursing home rates of use has produced a wave of perhaps predictable scandals. State Medicaid programs began to discourage nursing home use for those requiring relatively easy care while expanding home and community based services. At the same time, the private assisted-living industry expanded, absorbing an increasing share of the easier-care patients able to pay out of pocket for their care.[9] The result was a decline in nursing home occupancy and the closing of some marginal homes. The good news was that these shifts tended to break down the remaining invisible color barriers in access to blacks and shifted Medicaid recipients to better quality homes. As a result, rates of black use of nursing homes began for the first time to exceed white use (Smith et al. 2008).

The bad news is that marginal nursing homes in predominantly minority urban areas suffering occupancy problems began to fill beds with the previous occupants of state mental hospitals and prisons. For everyone, except neighborhoods and the homes' more traditional residents, it was a "win-win" solution. The more marginal urban homes could now fill their beds and break even. The hospital emergency rooms were relieved of having to admit as inpatients those who didn't belong and for whom payment would likely be denied. These "GOMERs" (Get Out of My Emergency Room patients), who had a central role in Samuel Shem's classic novel *House of God*, some of whom had medical problems that justified admission but could not be cured, have long been the bane of the existence of emergency room physicians (Shem 1995). For the individual admitted to a nursing home under these circumstances, it offered a relative paradise. The alternative was the street, jail, or a crowded, understaffed, bare-bone homeless shelter. Even for the state, responsible for paying the bill, it represented a winning proposition. The federal Medicaid match would make it less costly than the prison or even in many cases a homeless shelter option.

The transformation of these homes, however, could have a disas-

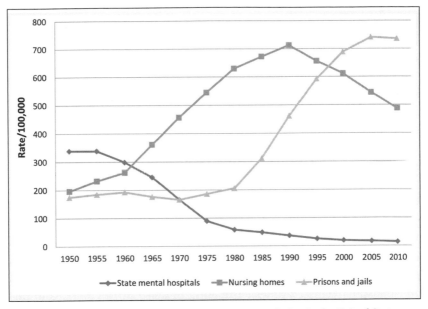

Figure 1. Rates of institutionalization per 100,000 population in the United States, 1950–2010

Sources. Population: US Bureau of the Census 2012; State and county mental hospital census: Substance Abuse and Mental Health Administration 2008, 43, and for 2010, Torrey 2012, 23; Nursing home census: US Bureau of the Census 2012; Prison and jail census 1950–1980 (with mid-decade estimates interpolated from the decennial census): Cahalan 1986; and for 1985–2010, Bureau of Justice Statistics 2011, 3.

trous impact on surrounding neighborhoods. In Chicago, for example, which had a particularly large excess capacity of nursing home beds bordering black areas of the city, local communities protested. These homes were not local community institutions. They were ones acquired by remote, privately held chains whose facilities in white areas got good ratings by the federal Medicare Nursing Home Compare Rating and whose homes in these black communities got abysmal ratings (Lowenstein 2009). Indeed, instead of being anchors of stability for these communities, they have often accelerated their decay. The new nursing home residents were increasingly parolees, sex offenders, drug addicts, and psychiatric patients. In some of these homes the majority of residents were under sixty-five. One home had more than 190 "walk offs" in a year. Nursing home residents are free to leave anytime they want to, unlike prison inmates and some psychiatric hospital patients. One typical protocol for the discharge of drug and alcohol or psychiatric patients in a nursing home is to count them as a discharge only if they fail to return in forty-eight hours. The local community is on its own in dealing with the problems caused by the "walk offs."

The elderly residents of these homes have to deal with all the problems that remain in those admissions of this type. In most cases there aren't any. In some, they have proved fatal. "Ivory Jacks had Alzheimer's disease, but that wasn't what killed him. At 77 he was smashed in the face with a clock radio as he lay in his bed at a south side nursing home. Jackson's roommate—a mentally ill man 30 years younger—was charged with the killing" (C. K. Johnson 2009, 1). "A nursing home dinner of pot roast, green beans and potatoes may have proved fatal to a 72 year old west side man. It wasn't the meal that killed him, prosecutors say, but a fellow resident of the Columbus Park Nursing Center who was furious that he had sneaked into his room and stolen his grub. His murderer had served prison time for drug offenses and had a history of abusing staff" (Janssen 2009). The point of these stories is to again underscore the racial disparities of the statistics in Figure 1, on both black communities and patients. One can't help believing that the race of the community and victims helped quiet the trouble in a way that would not have been tolerated in more affluent white communities.

Marching On

Yet those that had seen the glory continued to march on. For all the backsliding, the system did change. Medicare, the gift of that struggle, survives. The march to the Promised Land continues, guided by the same simple idea that propelled both the civil rights movement and Medicare's creation: "We are all in this together."

Nations as well as families respond to the same basic human instinct and look after each other. That same instinct produced the formation of the Knights and Daughters of Tabor by freed slaves that led to the construction of Taborian Hospital in Mound Bayou, Mississippi, which would spawn the modern civil rights movement. It would lead to the creation of similar mutual aid societies by nineteenth-century immigrant groups and the creation of arrangements for caring for members that became ill or incapacitated. That same idea led the Chicago Black Panthers to set up a free clinic on the devastated West Side of Chicago in 1969. In other nations, less fragmented by racial, ethnic, and class divides, it led to the development of national social insurance systems that would assure universal coverage. The United States, however, during the formative years of its health system's development, followed a different path. It led to a fragmented private insurance system and reluctant public subsidies to support care for those unable to afford such private protection and, to a large extent, continues to follow this path.

At the time of the passage of Medicare, it was assumed by all those implementing the program that it would soon expand to provide universal coverage (Oberlander and Marmor 2015). Medicaid, a last-minute addition to the package, they assumed, was just another substandard state program for the poor that would fade away. It didn't. Medicaid rather than Medicare now serves as the major vehicle for expanding health insurance coverage under the Affordable Care Act. In the wake of the complexity and cost of implementing the Affordable Care Act, many ask: "Why not Medicare for all?" (Seidman 2015, 909). Public opinion polls generally express a preference for such an option. Most hospital administrators and practicing physicians would prefer it (although many fewer would say so publicly, fearing retribution from the plethora of health plans they must negotiate contracts with in order to survive). What happened?

None of the explanations for why this didn't happen are very satisfying. True, the program as originally negotiated with hospitals and medicine resulted in rapidly rising costs that have proved difficult to correct (Starr 2015). True, the generous benefits to seniors created an entrenched special interest group fearful that any expansion to others would threaten their own benefits (Schlesinger 2015). True, these two impediments resulted in the replacement of Medicare by the traditional welfare model, Medicaid, as the vehicle for expanding coverage, most notably in the Affordable Care Act (Thompson 2015). Certainly "Medicare for All" has missed many opportunities in the past half century. Its critics now argue that we have to move on from where we are, and that's just the way it is (see, for example, Pollack 2015). The system has indeed found ingenious ways to "quiet trouble."

Yet battles were won in the struggle to assure an end to separate and unequal care. They were won in a time that had even more ingenious and sinister ways to "quiet trouble." They were won in a health system and political order even more resistant to change, in which the pervasive conventional wisdom was that, however irrational and unjust, "it was just the way things were." It began in part with the moral appeal posed in Gunnar Myrdal's widely read book The *American Dilemma*, that separate could never be equal and could never be reconciled with the fundamental American belief in fairness and equal opportunity (Myrdal 1944). That conclusion, referencing Myrdal's book, was echoed in the Supreme Court's *Brown* decision a decade later. At the height of the civil rights movement in the United States the logic of solidarity broke the mold of a health system created in its formative years. It produced a universal system of social insurance for the nation's elderly that covered their health care. It said, at least for our seniors, we are all in it together, and we look after each other. It said there can be no distinctions on the basis of race or income in access to care.

Why were those battles won, and what lessons can be learned from those victories? They involved no magic, no clever sleights of hand. Health care was just a little bit closer to achieving three necessary conditions for such a transformation.

1. UNIVERSAL REQUIREMENTS

Medicare Title VI guidelines required that race could not play any role in what facility people used, what bed they occupied, or how they were treated. It didn't try to persuade, educate, or offer people choices. It was a structural, system-wide solution. No exceptions. Giving organizations or individuals the "freedom of choice" to segregate, as far as OEHO inspectors saw it, was surrender. Hospitals and individuals, of course, were "free to choose" not to participate. Medicare just wouldn't pick up the tab. For those that did choose to participate, they would "all be in it together."

That rock-hard insistence eliminated uncertainty. For hospitals choosing to participate, there would be no white flight, and patients would have little concern about poorer care or personal safety. "Everything will be fine, the times are changing," the physicians could reassure their hospitalized patients. It was a self-fulfilling prophecy. A system that eliminates freedom of choice can't be gamed by one group at the expense of another. The same approach had been successfully used earlier by presidential executive orders to desegregate the armed services, Veteran's Administration facilities, Social Security Administration offices, and US Postal Service. Medicare's implementation just demonstrated it was possible to extend that approach beyond the boundaries of the agencies of the federal government.

2. NO MISSION, NO MARGIN

There has always been something more important than race, religion, ethnicity, gender, social class, or even political ideology in the United States, and it has usually been money. All individuals and institutions worry about their margin—income has to cover expenses. "No margin, no mission," as executives of voluntary hospital systems are fond of saying. Title VI Medicare certification, however, turned this on its head and, in effect, said, "No mission, no margin." The enforcement of Title VI in the implementation of Medicare demonstrated for the first time the power of the federal government to alter the mission of private institutions. It transformed hospitals by giving them a strong financial incentive to do so. In general, the parts of the health system that have remained the most racially and economically segregated and for which there are the largest racial and economic disparities in the access and quality of care (for example, nursing homes, home care, and some forms of specialty care) are those with the largest differences in what providers are paid in caring for the affluent as opposed to the indigent.

3. GRASSROOTS TROUBLE

Indeed, "the system only changes to quiet trouble." Change happens when there is sustained grassroots pressure for it. It was the grassroots pressure that made the hospital desegregation effort work. There would have been no civil rights laws or Title VI guidelines without it. Most likely, there would not have been a Medicare program at all. Medicare, at least in terms of how it was implemented, was the gift of the civil rights movement. Certainly it was aided by the brilliant legislative maneuvering of President Johnson and by the astute persistence of Secretary Gardner, Robert Ball, and Wilbur Cohen in its implementation. The diverse assortment of volunteers that rallied to the civil rights movement's cause, however, carried the day. They became the only public interest guardian at the gate in Medicare's implementation. Other aspects (how much hospitals would be paid and what quality standards they would have to meet to be eligible for such payments) was, to a large extent, delegated to the providers of services. In these areas, Medicare followed the classic model of regulatory capture by an industry.

What standards they would have to meet to be Title VI compliant was, however, captured by the civil rights movement. It was only in this area that Medicare was captured, not by the industry being regulated but by a social movement seeking to transform it. The combined power of a uniform standard, the purse, and grassroots activism made the transformation of health care, however incomplete, possible.

Yet disparities in health and access to care, carefully tracked for the first time over the last two decades, haven't moved that much. Some of the old "it's just the way things are" and less of the "we're all in it together" ethic that drove the original passage of Medicare has crept in to political and health professional debates. There are, however, some hopeful signs.

First, the goals of eliminating racial and economic disparities are now broadly shared, and all the goals of health care providers are now far better aligned with eliminating racial and economic disparities. Health care providers view racial, ethnic, and economic differences in care and health far differently today than they did at the beginning of the civil rights era. Although few would acknowledge it, this change was largely the result of persistent federal pressure. Most dismissed such differences then as the product of differences in behavior and genetics and not as something that providers or the nation as a whole had any responsibility to address. Title VI, Medicare, and Medicaid changed this. It changed the language used in describing such differences and shifted responsibility. Title VI prohibited providers receiving federal funds from treating patients differently because of their race or ethnicity ("disparate treatment") or engaging in seemingly racially neutral practices that adversely affected patients based on their race or ethnicity ("disparate impact").

Adopting the language of Title VI, racial and ethnic differences in health care treatment and health are now described as "disparities," implying that they are unfair and that providers and the nation as a whole have a moral and possibly legal responsibility to correct them. Indeed, the goal of eliminating such disparities is now almost universally embraced. Healthy People, a national public health collaborative planning effort, has set the elimination of disparities as its central goal for three decades, a goal embraced by presidents of both parties (US Department of Health and Human Services 2000, 1991; Department of Health and Human Services 2010). For the last decade, Congress has mandated that a national annual report on disparities in quality of care be completed with the goal of eliminating them (Agency for Healthcare Research and Quality 2012). The two bastions of the health care establishment, the AMA and AHA, which civil rights activists challenged in the 1960s, albeit belatedly, now collaborate with similar groups in efforts to reduce disparities. The AMA has even formally apologized to the NMA for its past conduct in obstructing black physician access to membership and hospital privileges and has joined it as a partner in a Commission to End Health Care Disparities (Commission to End Health Care Disparities 2010). The AHA, many of whose members did not distinguish themselves in this earlier period in assuring equity in access, has now joined with other hospital groups in an effort to eliminate disparities by: (1) increasing the collection of race, ethnicity, and language-preference data, (2) increasing the cultural competency training of physicians, and (3) increasing diversity in hospital governance and management (American Hospital Association 2014).

Are some of these professed commitments to eliminating disparities just paper assurances similar to those that some hospitals tried to get by with in the implementation of the Medicare program? Perhaps. More than a trillion in Medicare and Medicaid dollars—taxpayer dollars—now flow into our health system. Well-crafted Title VI guidelines and reporting requirements can and should assist the federal government in serving as a gatekeeper for these funds. The business case for providers to do more than just paper compliance, increasing market share and reducing malpractice risks, is straightforward.

Second, the Affordable Care Act (ACA), when it is fully implemented, will eliminate two major loopholes that have plagued Title VI certifications efforts: (1) it extends Title VI requirements to physicians and health plans receiving public funds and not just hospitals, and (2) it requires the collection and dissemination of data to monitor compliance. In addition, ACA restores the more recently lost private right of action (Watson 2012; Teitelbaum, Cartwright-Smith, and Rosenbaum 2012). Indeed, just expanding insurance coverage gets you closer to a "tipping point," when the "logic of solidarity" kicks in and one's own premium costs are shaped by the disparities in health and health care treatment of others. Also buried in the ACA is a provision (section 9007) that links nonprofit hospital tax exempt status to a triennial community health needs assessment and implementation strategy, potentially full of diverse community organizing and engagement efforts, trademarks of the civil rights movement (Rosenbaum 2013). Tax exemptions are dispensed to those who do work that embodies our moral commitments as a nation. Certainly the work of those institutions that demonstrate a commitment to the achievement of health equity should be high on the list.

Medicare and the civil rights reforms that accompanied it were gifts to the American people of a social movement in an all-too-brief period of national unity. A gift involves no expectation of getting anything directly in return. This was certainly the case for those who spontaneously chose to participate in civil rights movement direct actions, the black physicians and dentists who chose to challenge the hospital exclusions, and the many federal civil servants who chose to volunteer as compliance officers, accepting all the risks and long hours. Many paid a price for those decisions, and certainly most of those mentioned specifically in this book did. Yet most remembered this period as the happiest time in their lives. Their gift was one that no politician of whatever persuasion dares try to take away. The story about the tea party activist demanding that their conservative South Carolina congressman "keep his government hands off my Medicare" is not really that funny after all (Rucker 2009). You don't take away a gift, particularly one that is so important and wasn't really the government's anyway.

We are a long way from the Promised Land, and there will certainly be difficult days ahead. Yet, faced with far more intractable difficulties, the individuals and organizations described in this book produced a remarkable transformation. We have the power to heal.

Notes

Preface

1. Twin brother Woollcott was a "Freedom Rider" in the summer of 1961 and served time in the maximum security unit at the state penitentiary in Parchman, Mississippi. Sister Barbara was involved in the summer of 1965 tutoring students in Holly Springs, Mississippi, and doing voter registration. My mother, Nancy, with other Massachusetts friends, was jailed in the spring of 1964 for picketing outside the Sears Roebuck store in Williamston, North Carolina, which would not hire blacks. Faced with intransigence and blocked from any possibility of earning a livelihood, many were forced to leave. The Massachusetts group facilitating their show of support for the Williamston movement helped relocate to the Boston area many of the families of movement leaders. The price paid and the intractable bitterness of the conflict gets lost in the carefully packaged feel-good closure of most current accounts.

2. The PhD program in medical care organization in what was then the Bureau of Public Health Economics in the School of Public Health was the brainchild of medical care reformers Nathaniel Sinai, who had served on the staff of the Committee on the Cost of Medical Care in the early 1930s, and Seymour Axelrod, who assisted (former Michigan faculty member who later served as dean of their School of Social Work) Wilbur Cohen, undersecretary of HEW during the 1965–66 implementation of the Medicare program. The faculty that worked with the doctoral students, Ben Darsky, Charles Metzner, and Avedis Donabedian, were more traditional academics rather than public policy entrepreneurs, concerned with building a systematic body of knowledge. Their influence and elusive vision shaped all my subsequent efforts.

3. Later labeled HMOs and more recently "managed care," they were then "prepaid group practices." They were still considered "socialism" and an unethical form of medical practice by the American Medical Association and had yet to migrate from being the reform panacea of the left (most prepaid group practices had been set up by labor unions and attracted more liberal, reform-minded physicians) to the commercial insurance panacea of the right.

4. The suit, *Taylor v. White*, No. 90-3307 (E.D. Pa., amended complaint filed August 15, 1990), linked capital reimbursement policies and the failure to monitor civil rights compliance to marked disparities in black access to nursing homes. Concerned with protecting their interests, all three state nursing home associations joined with the Department of Welfare in defending against the suit. The seriousness of the access problems at the time, stimulated by the introduction of prospective payment for hospitals in both the Medicare and Medicaid programs, were abated by the introduction of similar financial incentives in Medicaid payments to nursing homes that discouraged the admission of patients in need of less intensive nursing care. This led to the growth of home- and community-based alternatives for Medicaid beneficiaries and the rapid growth of private assisted living developments. While marked disparities in the quality of nursing homes used by blacks as opposed to whites remain, the gross differences in access to nursing homes no longer exist (see Smith et al. 2008). The second suit, *Madison-Hughes v. Shalala*, No. 3-93-0046 (M.D. Tenn., filed January 19, 1993), tried to force HHS to collect data that could be used to enforce Title VI compliance. The suit was dismissed. The court concluded that if HHS didn't need to collect information on whether recipients of its funds were in compliance with Title VI in order to certify them in compliance, they were free not to do so. The absurdity of such an "Emperor's New Clothes" type of certification was obvious (or at least now public), and efforts to collect and analyze information initially through a federal interagency task force and subsequent reports from the Center for Medicare and Medicaid Services began, eventually being included in the requirements imposed on all participating providers and plans in the Affordable Care Act of 2010. These changes would have perhaps happened without the suits, but many interested in making such changes (including, apparently, the individual targets of these suits), welcomed them.

5. The interviews and other materials collected by the project are available in the David Barton Smith Hospital Segregation Files, Charles L. Blockson Afro-American Collection, Temple University Library. Many of the taped interviews were reviewed again in the production of this manuscript since most of the remarkable individuals I had the opportunity to interview are now deceased. I was particularly indebted to the encouragement of Sol Levine and David Mechanic, who helped direct the RWJ Investigator Program, providing much encouragement. The program continues to be a source of ideas and stimulation. The most recent was participating in the development of and providing a chapter in a collection published last year on the Medicare program for its fiftieth anniversary (Smith 2015a).

6. Barbara Berney, professor in the School of Public Health, Hunter College, has been a marvelous collaborator, and I have taken advantage of some of the interviews and materials her team has pulled together fleshing out the story in this book. I look forward to further assisting in the effort to translate

the story into a documentary film. Others participating in this effort include Anna Reid Jhirad, Dante James, Vanessa Burrows, and Madeline Gordon.

7. I am indebted to those who helped me to contribute to their projects: Thomas Oliver, *Guide to U.S. Health and Health Care Policy* (Smith 2014); Alan B. Cohen, David C. Colby, Keith A. Wailoo, and Julian E. Zelizer, *Medicare and Medicaid at 50* (Smith 2015a); and Ruqaiijah Yearby, *Health Matrix Journal of Law-Medicine Symposium* (Smith 2015b). Their encouragement and insights found their way into the pages of this book.

Chapter 1

1. Journalist T. R. Reid supplies a readable account of the contrast between the United States and other developed countries that embrace the logic of social solidarity when it comes to assuring universal protection to citizens (Reid 2010). Hoffman offers a fine historical account of rationing of health care in the United States largely along racial lines (Hoffman 2012). Quadagno provides a convincing account of the role race has played in the failures of Johnson's War on Poverty programs (Quadagno 1994). Stone fleshes out its role in the evolution of health insurance in the United States and its transformation from more inclusive community rating of premiums to a more experienced rating of premiums as a reflection of this lack of social solidarity (Stone 1993). The explanation for American exceptionalism, while typically cloaked in the rhetoric of individualism, free enterprise, and cultural conservatism, statistically appears more a product of its troubled racial history. The greater redistribution of wealth in European-style welfare states reflects public opinion survey results that attribute most poverty to misfortune, while similar surveys in the United States attribute poverty, disproportionately present in racial minorities, mostly to laziness (Alesina, Glaeser, and Sacerdote 2001).

2. As a model, the Mound Bayou Community Health Center (Now the Delta Health Center, Inc.) thrived despite state and federal political obstacles assuring local community control (the majority of the boards of federally funded health centers must be patients). These federally supported centers borrowed the model developed earlier to address the lack of access to health care for blacks in apartheid South Africa, and it spread across the United States winning broad bi-partisan support. In 2010 there were more than twelve hundred federally qualified community health centers operating more than eight thousand primary care delivery sites, caring for about twenty million patients, and the Affordable Care Act proposed funding for doubling these numbers over the next decade (Adashi, Geiger, and Fine 2010). The health center didn't stop just at writing prescriptions for food. They got involved in reintroducing food production in the Delta, organizing a farm co-op. For the first planting season they needed a backhoe and a couple of forty-horsepower tractors. They needed them right away, and the check

from the Ford Foundation to support these purchases had yet to arrive. Not to be thwarted, Geiger, the project's director, provided the money. "I said, OK, I'll stick it in the capital equipment budget—OEO never looks at that. Go out and buy the backhoe and tractors now. Then, when the Ford money comes, I'll repay the grant. They did. Of course that was the year OEO looked at the equipment budget. It turned out that these items had been stuck in the middle of the obstetric list. I found out when I got a deadpan call from someone at OEO asking me to describe what kind of deliveries we were planning" (Geiger 2015).

3. Robert L. Phillips, MD, interview with author in Greensboro, NC (David Barton Smith Hospital Segregation Files, 2015).

4. The account of Drew's death presented here summarizes the spellbinding, well-researched account by Spencie Love (Love 1996).

5. For all its limitations, the Hill-Burton Act of 1946 did succeed in helping to equalize the supply of hospital beds available to blacks compared to whites as Thomas documents (Thomas 2011).

6. Ms. Mattie Gadson taped interview with author, Philadelphia, 1996 (David Barton Smith Hospital Segregation Files, 2015).

7. Gadson interview.

8. "Cicero Race Riot of 1951," *Wikipedia*, Wikimedia Foundation. Last modified October 25, 2014. *en.wikipedia.org/wiki/Cicero_race_riot_of_1951*.

9. Quentin Young, MD, taped interview with author in Chicago, June 1997 (David Barton Smith Hospital Segregation Files, 2015).

10. Quentin Young interview.

11. This account relies for the most part on an interview with Dr. Young and documents that he supplied.

12. Quentin Young interview.

13. Quentin Young interview.

14. Paul Cornely, MD, taped interview with author 1990 (David Barton Smith Hospital Segregation Files, 2015).

15. Quentin Young interview.

Chapter 2

1. This section relies mostly on the remarkable story pulled together by David T. Beito and Linda Royster Beito on T. R. M. Howard's life (Beito and Beito 2009).

2. Mound Bayou had a long history of black self-sufficiency beginning with its founding by former slaves of Joseph Emory Davis (brother of Confederate president Jefferson Davis), Isaiah Montgomery, and Benjamin Green, as a place of refuge for blacks in 1887 and the nation's first all-black town. Booker T. Washington recognized it as a model example of self-help and entrepreneurial advancement. In a twist of irony, Theodore Roosevelt Mason Howard was named after the first president to invite a black man, Booker T.

Washington, to a meal at the White House. During the civil rights era Mound Bayou would serve as one of the two birthplaces of federally supported community health centers. The number of federally supported health centers has grown to more than twelve hundred, serving about twenty million people across the nation and targeted for substantial increases under the Affordable Care Act (Adashi, Geiger, and Fine 2010).

3. For a well written summary of the Sovereignty Commissions activities, see Bowers 2010. Most of the documentation is now available online and provides an eerie narrative of its own. See *mdah.state.ms.us/arrec/digital_archives/sovcom*.

4. I have summarized the story of Dr. Hereford's life here largely making use of the autobiography jointly authored by Dr. Hereford and Jack Ellis (Hereford and Ellis 2011) and through subsequent contacts with both authors in preparing this section of the manuscript.

5. According to my telephone interview with Dr. Hereford in 2015, one of the physicians, a recent medical school graduate, had just set up his practice and was concerned about the repercussions it might have on his ability to get patient referrals and other help from white colleagues necessary for a livelihood. The other, an older practitioner with a long-established practice, was perhaps reluctant to offend white colleagues with whom he had a well-established, comfortable relationship. In Huntsville, as in most other communities, black physicians' involvement as civil rights activists was limited to a minority and, in the case of Huntsville, a minority of one. Just as in other communities, black dentists were less constrained since their practices were less dependent on their relationships with white colleagues. Indeed, Hereford's key activist ally was John L. Cashin Jr., DDS. Cashin was part of a long family tradition of civil rights agitators. His grandfather had served as a radical Republican legislator during Reconstruction in Alabama, and he would later run as a third-party candidate for governor against Wallace in 1970. (Dentist Reginald Hawkins had several years earlier run a campaign for governor in North Carolina.) Cashin's daughter, Sheryll, would get an early start, arrested at the age of four months with her mother in a sit-in in Huntsville. Graduating summa cum laude from Vanderbilt University in 1984, she received her JD at Harvard Law School with honors and clerked for Thurgood Marshall, one of the last to have this opportunity. She is currently a professor of law at Georgetown and a forceful advocate for an end to de facto segregation (see, for example, Cashin 2014).

6. According to Sonnie Hereford III in a telephone interview with the author in 2015, Sonnie Hereford IV now serves as chief of operations for the army at Huntsville.

7. Reginald Hawkins taped interview with author in Charlottesville, 2000 (David Barton Smith Hospital Segregation Files, 2015).

8. In a lively interview with Reginald Hawkins in 2000 at a diner near Johnson C. Smith College in Charlotte, constantly interrupted by well-wishers, Dr.

Hawkins fondly remembered helping to spirit Thurgood Marshall past threatening local vigilantes to a South Carolina court—where one of the cases was argued that would become part of the Brown decision—from Charlotte in the back of a hearse. The interracial group of lawyers with Hawkins all sat on the floor of the black funeral director's hearse, laughed, told off-color stories, and passed around Marshall's bottle of good scotch. Dr. Hawkins seemed to feed off the adrenalin rush of these memories.

9. Reginald Hawkins interview.

10. On the same front page of the *Charlotte Observer* announcing the decision of Presbyterian to integrate was a separate article announcing their plan to build a new wing, presumably with the assistance of Hill-Burton funds that would include only private rooms.

11. Reginald Hawkins interview.

12. Both the symbolism and substance of this shift in editorship was profound. Booker T. Washington, director of the Tuskegee Institute, was the author of the 1895 "Atlanta Compromise," which proposed that blacks seek separate, independent development and not challenge white supremacy or segregation. The basic precepts of this "compromise" were never directly challenged during Kenney's tenure as editor.

13. Cobb helped with any who shared the vision of ending segregation and not just former Howard students. For example, as described in Chapter 1, he worked closely with Jack Geiger and other University of Chicago students in helping to document the problems that medical school applicants and patients faced.

14. In order to avoid being forced to integrate their white medical schools or to bear the expense of establishing black ones, some southern states, such as Georgia and Alabama, established scholarships programs for black state residents to attend the nation's two historically black medical schools, Howard and Meharry. Both schools through their graduates played a central role in the civil rights desegregation campaigns but were also beneficiaries of Jim Crow policies.

15. Paul Cornely interview.

16. This account was derived from an interview with Dr. Watts in 1996 with the subsequent assistance of his daughter C. Eileen Welch while this book was being written in 2015.

17. Charles Watts, MD, taped interview with author, Durham, NC August 28, 1996 (David Barton Smith Hospital Segregation Files, 2015).

18. Charles Watts interview.

19. Charles Watts interview.

20. The maternal grandfather of Dr. Watts's wife, Constance—Dr. Moore—had founded Lincoln Hospital in 1901 with some funding from the Duke family. He served as its superintendent until his death in 1920. The options for black surgeons then were limited, and Dr. Watts was one of the more fortunate. Dr. Watts's grandson Dr. Babu G. Welch followed a similar path, graduating from

Howard Medical School in 1997. Facing few of the barriers his grandfather faced, he is a board-certified neurosurgeon at the University of Texas Southwestern Medical Center and medical director of their Neurosurgery Ambulatory Clinic and Microvascular Laboratory.

21. Charles Watts interview.
22. Charles Watts interview.
23. Charles Watts interview.
24. The glamour of the US Open with the likes of Tiger Woods left conditions in the segregated black community that continues to supply much of the service staff of Pinehurst unimproved. They seemingly live within the boundaries of a luxurious resort community but still apparently can't get city water or sewage (Chambers 2008).
25. Charles Watts interview.
26. Charles Watts interview.
27. George Simkins Jr., DDS, tape-recorded interview with author in Greensboro, North Carolina, May 3, 1996 (David Barton Smith Hospital Segregation Files, 2015).
28. George Simkins interview.
29. George Simkins interview.

Chapter 3

1. The account presented here summarizes the remarkable story told by Taylor Branch (Branch 1988, 352–78).
2. These ratios have remained essentially unchanged despite the preferences of the electorates in most southern states to support the reduction in federal spending (see Pear 1996, Wikipedia 2015). All the states in the former Jim Crow South have chosen not to expand Medicaid coverage under the Affordable Care Act despite the benefits in expanding coverage to lower-income residents and the financial benefits this would offer both hospitals and physicians of their states (Kaiser Family Foundation 2015b).
3. Charles Johnson, taped interview with author, Durham, NC, 1996 (David Barton Smith Hospital Segregation Files, 2015).
4. The account of the desegregation of the hospitals in Jackson, Mississippi, was pieced together from the documents available online from the Sovereignty Commission files made available by the Mississippi Department of Archives and History; see *mdah.state.ms.us/arrec/digital_archives/sovcom*.
5. Quentin Young interview.
6. Quentin Young interview.
7. Harold Bettis, interview with author, Greensboro, NC, 1996 (David Barton Smith Hospital Segregation Files, 2015).
8. Joseph Califano, telephone interview with author June 24, 2015 (David Barton Smith Hospital Segregation Files, 2015).
9. There is the widely accepted myth that, with all the difficulties in passing and

implementing the Affordable Care Act in more recent times, the legislative process was more functional in the 1960s than today, with a greater degree of mutual respect, trust, and bipartisan collaboration. As Julian Zelizer demonstrates in a review, one could make the case that it was even more dysfunctional (Zelizer 2015).

10. US District Court, Northern District of Illinois, Eastern Division at Chicago, Civil Case 61C1659, *James William Webb Jr. and Andrew Webb, minors, by James R. Webb, their parent and next friend, et al. v. Board of Education, City of Chicago.*

11. As noted by Joseph Califano is his interview with the author on June 24, 2015, those attending the signing included representatives from the Jewish American and Italian American communities concerned about fairness in immigration policies for Soviet Jews and southern Italians, and no one anticipated its more long-term impact. In terms of electoral politics, even the new solid Republican South seemed destined to collapse from the resulting racial and ethnic demographic shifts (see, for example, Raines 2015).

12. Joseph Califano, interview with author, July 24, 2015.

Chapter 4

1. Telephone conversation between Peter Libassi and author, August 1, 2015 (David Barton Smith Hospital Segregation Files, 2015).

2. Telephone interview with Ted Marmor on April 8, 2014 (David Barton Smith Hospital Segregation Files).

3. Derrick Bell's law school text on civil rights law survived six editions (Bell 2010). He was a provocative, creative, and prolific writer. Bell later despaired of progress in federal enforcement of civil rights and even the contribution of the *Brown* decision to educational equity (Bell 1987, 2004). Yet he never completed the circle back to Booker T. Washington's Atlanta Compromise position and, despite his barbed critiques, grudgingly held out hope for racial integration.

4. Peter Libassi, telephone interview by author on August 1, 2016 (David Barton Smith Hospital Segregation Files, 2015).

5. Notes from follow-up telephone interview with Peter Libassi by author on August 10, 2015 (David Barton Smith Hospital Segregation Files, 2015).

6. Ted Marmor telephone interview with author April 8, 2014 (David Barton Smith Hospital Segregation Files, 2015).

7. The general operating principle in organizing Title VI compliance efforts was to avoid, for the sake of the organizations involved and the efficiency of the federal effort, having more than one agency responsible for compliance. Hospitals were recipients of two kinds of public funding: the Public Health Service's Hill-Burton Program for construction and the Social Security Administration's Medicare Program for services provided to Medicare

beneficiaries. The Public Health Service was assigned the responsibility for Title VI compliance in both programs.

8. Robert Ball, telephone conversation with author, September 1998 (David Barton Smith Hospital Segregation Files, 2015).

9. Frank Weil, taped interview with author, OCR, Washington, DC, May 26, 1995 (David Barton Smith Hospital Segregation Files, 2015).

10. Frank Weil interview.

11. Frank Weil interview.

12. Frank Weil interview.

13. Peter Libassi, telephone interview with author on August 1, 2015 (David Barton Smith Hospital Segregation Files).

14. In a 2015 telephone interview by the author, Joseph Califano had no recollection of the interchange with Libassi but faced many more pressing matters and acknowledged that Medicare's implementation that year got little of his attention. It was something best left to HEW officials and the hospitals who were entrusted in making it work. Although the exact date was uncertain, the interchange was still a vivid recollection for Libassi, based on my telephone conversation with him on August 1, 2015 (David Barton Smith Hospital Segregation Files 2015).

15. There is no written record of these impromptu remarks, but they have become one of King's most often quoted lines. Quentin Young, who was chairman of the Medical Committee for Human Rights that year and in the audience, recalled the words (see Moore 2013).

16. Ruth McVay, taped interview by author in OCR offices in Washington, DC, June 7, 1996 (David Barton Smith Hospital Segregation Files, 2015).

17. Julian Suttle, administrator of Social Security in Montgomery Alabama during the 1960s, notes from telephone interview with Barbara Berney, January 8, 2013 (David Barton Smith Hospital Segregation Files, 2015).

18. Ruth McVay interview.

19. Julian Suttle interview.

20. Frank Weil interview.

21. Frank Weil interview.

22. Frank Weil interview.

23. Frank Weil interview.

24. J. W. Pinkston, interview with author in Atlanta, June 10, 1996 (David Barton Smith Hospital Segregation Files, 2015).

25. Peter Libassi, telephone interview with author, August 10, 2015.

26. Charles Watts interview 1996.

27. Ruth McVay interview.

28. Ruth McVay interview.

29. Frank Weil interview.

30. Ruth McVay interview.

31. Libassi vividly remembered this as a part of the June 15 meeting with the hospitals. It was not in the transcripts of Johnson's remarks, but such ad libs,

particularly an earthy one that aides may have felt not in keeping with his stature as a world leader, might well not have been included.

32. The only possible exception would be for admission for elective procedures, but admissions for elective procedures can be managed and scheduled. They would not create any life-threatening access problems to hospital care.

33. Ted Marmor, telephone interview with author, April 8, 2014 (David Barton Smith Hospital Segregation Files, 2015).

Chapter 5

1. I am indebted to Eric Delisle, historian in the Historian's Office at the Social Security Administration for digging through Commissioner Ball's correspondence files for these letters, which reveal much about Commissioner Ball and how he handled both the internal organizational problems and external pressures related to Title VI enforcement.

2. Peter Libassi, interview with author, August 10, 2015.

3. Susan Chapman, taped interview with author in 1995 in Philadelphia (David Barton Smith Hospital Segregation Files, 2015).

4. Earl Wert, MD, interview with author in Mobile, AL, May 7, 1998 (David Barton Smith Hospital Segregation Files, 2015).

5. E. C. Bramlett Jr., interview by author in 1998. Notes of interview are available in the David Barton Smith Hospital Segregation Files, Blockson Collection, Temple University Library, Philadelphia.

6. No records of the investigation into Dr. Cowsert's death apparently exist in the Mobile Police Department files. A Freedom of Information Act request to the FBI indicated that they as well have no record of such an investigation although one was apparently requested by OEHO. A similar Freedom of Information Act request of the Department of Health and Human Services indicated that all the working files of OEHO that would have been involved in their dispute with the Mobile Infirmary have long since been shredded as required by federal regulations. The entire critical year of correspondence of Congressman Jack Edwards (D, AL), who was active that year in advocating the Mobile Infirmary's case, is missing from his correspondence files turned over to the archive at the University of Southern Alabama. The record of the autopsy of Dr. Cowsert was apparently destroyed in a flood. Mobile is indeed a city that knows how to keep its secrets.

7. The description of the subsequent campaign largely summarizes some of the detailed and riveting account provided by Anderson and Pickering in *Confronting the Color Line: The Broken Promise of the Civil Rights Movement in Chicago* (Anderson and Pickering 1986).

8. Quentin Young interview.

9. Quentin Young interview.

10. Reginald Hawkins interview.

11. Charles Johnson interview.

12. Bobby Childers, taped telephone interview with Vanessa Burrows (David Barton Smith Hospital Segregation Files, 2015).
13. Ruth McVay interview.
14. Ruth McVay interview.
15. Leon Rodriquez, conversation with author, OCR offices in Washington, DC, April 22, 2014.
16. Leon Panetta, of course, survived his first and most humiliating job in the federal bureaucracy. He served as a Democratic congressman from California before returning in the Clinton administration as director of OMB and then as White House chief of staff. He returned during the Obama administration, serving as director of the Central Intelligence Agency and then as secretary of defense. Overseeing, as CIA director, drone attacks on Al-Qaeda leaders and the death of Osama Bin Laden, he had certainly managed to overcome his role as the passive, unknowing victim of Nixon's southern strategy.

Chapter 6

1. Representative Bobby Rush, transcript of interview with Barbara Berney, Chicago, July 2015, 8 (David Barton Smith Hospital Segregation Files, 2015).
2. Gadson interview 1996.
3. 42 USC § 1395dd, the Emergency Medical Treatment and Active Labor Act (EMTALA) was passed in 1986 as part of the Consolidated Budget Reconciliation Act (COBRA). It requires "participating hospitals" (those contracted to provide services to Medicare beneficiaries) to evaluate and treat medical emergencies regardless of citizenship, legal status, or ability to pay. It's a patchwork and inadequate solution for those lacking health insurance but one that has prevented indiscriminate dumping of patients critically needing care. Hospitals object to it as an "unfunded mandate," but none, just as in the case with the Title VI requirements, have chosen to terminate their participation in the Medicare program.
4. The willingness of hospitals to force this issue, of course, depends on their own financial needs and their relative negotiating power over physicians. The more dominant a hospital system is in its local market, the more willing the system is to force this issue. The growth of hospital systems through mergers and acquisitions increases their bargaining power to impose such requirements.
5. Fred Shuttlesworth was the ultimate street fighter, and this succinctly elegant assessment was one made in a visit to Coatesville, Pennsylvania, in 1999. The last survivor of the four ministers founding the SCLC in 1957, he was known by civil rights activists as "the Wild Man from Birmingham" and the key to the success of that campaign. His home was dynamited. When he tried to have his children integrate an all-white school in 1957, he was beaten by Klan members with bicycle chains and brass knuckles. When examined by a doctor for the resulting head wounds, who marveled that he had survived

without serious injury, he replied, "Doctor, the Lord knew I lived in a hard town, so he gave me a hard head." In the 2007 celebration of the anniversary of "Bloody Sunday" (the beating of civil rights marchers on the Edmund Pettus Bridge in Selma, Alabama, on March 7, 1965), then senator Barack Obama pushed Shuttlesworth's wheelchair across this same bridge. In 2009 Reverend Shuttlesworth attended, as the guest of honor in an audience of six thousand, a live public telecast of the swearing in of Barack Obama as president. He died at age eighty-nine in Birmingham in 2011 (Nordheimer 2011).

6. Sam Eichold, MD, taped interview with author, Mobile, AL, 1998 (David Barton Smith Hospital Segregation Files, 2015).

7. Howard Bennett, taped interview by author, Washington, DC, 1995 (David Barton Smith Hospital Segregation Files, 2015).

8. The Medicare and Medicaid law prohibited payments to state hospitals for the long-term mentally ill. Acute care hospitals and nursing homes have always cared for some mentally ill patients, but the question was, at what point did the proportion of mentally ill patients make a facility, in effect, an institution for the mentally ill and ineligible for payment? The financial incentives, for facilities and states to stray into the gray were and are substantial.

9. New Medicaid payments to nursing homes in many states shifted to Resource Utilization Group (RUG) payments during the 1990s. Similar to the earlier introduction of Diagnostic Related Group (DRG) payments to hospitals in the 1980s it created a disincentive to treat those not needing more intensive care and helped spawn the growth of alternative less costly settings such as home- and community-based services and assisted living (see, for example, Smith 2003).

Bibliography

Adashi, Ely Y., H. Jack Geiger, and Michael D. Fine. 2010. "Health Care Reform and Primary Care—the Growing Importance of the Community Health Center." *New England Journal of Medicine* 362 (22): 2047–50.

Agency for Healthcare Research and Quality. 2012. "National Healthcare Disparities Report 2011." *www.ahrq.gov/research/findings/nhqrdr/nhdr11/nhdr11.pdf.*

Alesina, Alberto, Edward Glaeser, and Bruce Sacerdote. 2001. "Why Doesn't the United States Have a European-Style Welfare State?" *Brookings Papers on Economic Activity* 2: 187–277.

Alexander, Michelle. 2012. *The New Jim Crow: Mass Incarceration in the Age of Color Blindness.* New York: New Press.

Almond, Douglas V., Kenneth Y. Chay, and Michael Greenstone. 2008. "The Civil Rights Act of 1964, Hospital Desegregation and Black Infant Mortality in Mississippi." Working Paper 07-04, Columbia University Department of Economics. December. New York. 1–24. *papers.ssrn.com/s013/papers.cfm?abstract_id=961021.*

American College of Surgeons. 1920. "Hospital Standardization." *Surgery, Gynecology and Obstetrics* 30: 641–47.

American Hospital Association. 2014. "Eliminating Racial and Ethnic Disparities." American Hospital Association. *www.equityofcare.org.*

Anderson, Alan B., and George W. Pickering. 1986. *Confronting the Color Line: The Broken Promise of the Civil Rights Movement in Chicago.* Athens: University of Georgia Press.

Ansell, David A. 2011. *County: Life, Death and Politics at Chicago's Public Hospital.* Chicago: Academy of Chicago Publishers.

Atlanta Daily World. 1947. "Ask Bias End at Hines Hospital." *Atlanta Daily World,* October 24, 1.

———. 1958. "Magazine Terms Chicago Worst Segregated Big City in U.S." *Atlanta Daily World,* September 17, 1.

Ball, Robert. 1966a. "The First 60 Days of Medicare." *Journal of the National Medical Association* 58 (6): 475–79.

———. 1966b. Letter to Senator Richard Russell, August 31. In Robert Ball

Correspondence files, Social Security Administration Archives. Baltimore: Social Security Administration.

———. 1966c. Memo from Robert Ball on Assuring Title VI Compliance before Signing Hospital Agreements October 25. In Robert Ball Correspondence files, Social Security Administration Archives. Baltimore: Social Security Administration.

Banta, Parks M. 1961. Memorandum from Parks M. Banta, General Counsel, HEW to the Secretary. Harris Wofford Papers. Boston: John F. Kennedy Library.

Beito, David T., and Linda Royster Beito. 2009. *Black Maverick: T. R. M. Howard's Fight for Civil Rights and Economic Power*. Champaign: University of Illinois Press.

Bell, Derrick A. 1966. Bell, Derrick A. 1966. *Memorandum to Robert Owen, Special Assistant to the Attorney General on Title VI: Notices of Hearings to Five Hospitals Refusing to Comply December*. Office Files of Douglas Cater, Box 14. Austin, TX: Lyndon Baines Johnson Library.

———. 1987. *And We Are Not Saved: The Elusive Quest for Racial Justice*. New York: Basic Books.

———. 2004. *Silent Covenant: Brown v. Board of Education and the Unfulfilled Hopes of Racial Reform*. New York: Oxford University Press.

———. 2010. *Race, Racism and American Law*. 6th ed. Waltham, MA: Wolters Kluwer.

Berkowitz Edward D. 1995. *Mr. Social Security: The Life of Wilbur J. Cohen*. Lawrence: University Press of Kansas.

Berman, Larry. 1981. "Chapter 6. Johnson and the White House Staff." In *Exploring the Johnson Years*, edited by Robert A. Devine, 187–213. Austin: University of Texas Press.

Berney, Barbara. 2015. "Interview Clip with Peter Libassi." Last modified July 17, 2015. *www.blbfilmproductions.com/about-the-film.html*.

Bernstein, Leon. 1976. "Conversation with Leon Bernstein by David Smith, Office of Research and Statistics, Social Security Administration." September.

Bowers, Rick. 2010. *Spies of Mississippi: The True Story of the Spy Network That Tried to Destroy the Civil Rights Movement*. Washington, DC: National Geographic.

Branch, Taylor. 1988. *Parting the Waters: America in the King Years 1954–63*. New York: Simon and Schuster.

Broom, Dick. 2002. "The First ICU: The Earliest Critically Ill Patients Found Intensive Care at UNC." *UNC Medical Center Public Relations Office*, University of North Carolina Medical Center. Press Packet.

Bryant, Farris. 1966. *Memorandum to the President, May*. White House Central Files. Austin, TX: Lyndon Baines Johnson Library.

Bureau of Justice Statistics. 2011. "Correctional Population in the United States 2010." *Bureau of Justice Statistics Bulletin*, December, 1–31.

Cahalan, Margaret Werner. 1986. *Historical Correction Statistics in the United States 1850–1984*. Rockville, MD: Westat.

Caldwell, Earl. 1971. "The Panthers: Dead or Regrouping." *New York Times*, March 1, 1, 16.

Califano, Joseph A. 1981. *Governing America: An Insider's Report from the White House and the Cabinet*. New York: Simon and Schuster.

———. 1991. *The Triumph and Tragedy of Lyndon Johnson: The White House Years*. New York: Simon and Schuster.

———. 2014. "The Movie 'Selma' Has a Glaring Flaw." *Washington Post*, January 7. *www.washingtonpost.com/opinions/the-movie-selma-has-a-glaring-historical-inaccuracy/2014/12/26/70ad3ea2-8aa4-11e4-a085-34e9b9f09a58_story.html*.

———. 2015. YouTube Video. In *An Evening with Joe Califano*, edited by Bob Schieffer. Austin, TX: Lyndon Baines Johnson Library.

Caputo, Philip. 1969. "5,000 Mourners Walk Past Coffin of Hampton in Suburb." *Chicago Tribune*, December 10, 3.

Cashin, Sheryll D. 2014. *Place Not Race: A New Vision of Opportunity in America*. Boston: Beacon.

Cater, Douglas. 1966. Memorandum to the President, Report on Hospital Civil Rights Compliance Efforts in the South. Edited by White House Central File. Austin, TX: Lyndon Baines Johnson Library.

Celebrezze, Anthony. 1965. Letter from Anthony Celebrezze to Senator Harry Byrd. White House Central Files. Austin, TX: Lyndon Baines Johnson Library.

Center for Medicare and Medicaid Services. 2015. "Readmission Reduction Program." Center for Medicare and Medicaid Services. *www.cms.gov/Medicare/Medicare-Fee-for-Service-Payment/AcuteInpatientPPS/Readmissions-Reduction-Program.html*.

Centers for Disease Control. 2014. "Table 1. Number of Deaths, Death Rates and Age-Adjusted Rates, by Race and Sex: United States 1940, 1950, 1960 and 1980–2006." Last modified May 2, 2009. *www.disastercenter.com/cdc/Table_1_2006.html*.

Chambers, Julius. 2008. "Martin Luther King Celebratory Speech: Vermont Law School 2008." *Vermont Law Review* 33 (Fall): 131.

Chetty, Raj, Nathaniel Hendren, and Lawrence F. Katz. 2015. *The Effects of Exposure to Better Neighborhoods on Children: New Evidence from the Moving to Opportunity Experiment*. Cambridge, MA: Harvard University and the National Bureau of Economic Research.

Chicago Daily Defender. 1918. "Segregation of Race Patients Is Ordered." *Chicago Daily Defender*, February 2, 1.

———. 1960. "Chicago—Model of Segregation." *Chicago Daily Defender*, July 14, 12.

———. 1966. "Feud Brews Here between Negro Medics and HEW." *Chicago Daily Defender*, May 31, 44.

———. 1969. "Panthers Plan to Open Free Medical Clinic." *Chicago Daily Defender*, July 14, 3.

———. 1970. "Move to Halt Clinic's Closing." *Chicago Daily Defender*, February 11, 2.

Chicago Tribune. 1970a. "2 Panther Clinic Medics Oppose Licensing by City." *Chicago Tribune*, February 20, 3.

———. 1970b. "Move against Chicago Clinic." *Chicago Tribune*, January 21, A4.

Clarion Ledger. 1969. "Baptist to Become Eligible for Medicare." *(Jackson, MS) Clarion Ledger*, April 9, 1.

Cobb, W. Montague. 1947. *Bulletin of the Medico-Chirugical Society of the District of Columbia* 4 (7): 3, 8, 10.

———. 1951. "Surgery and the Negro Physician: Some Parallels in Background." *Journal of the National Medical Association* 43: 148.

———. 1953. "The National Program of the NAACP." *Journal of the National Medical Association* 45 (5): 333–39.

———. 1954. "The Seventeenth of May." *Journal of the National Medical Association* 46: 269.

———. 1957. "Editorial: A Golden Opportunity." *Journal of the National Medical Association* 49 (1): 53.

———. 1961. "Chicago Physicians Sue for Admission to Hospital Staffs." *Journal of the National Medical Association* 53 (2): 198–99.

———. 1962. "Executive Procedure without Effect in Hospital Area." *Journal of the National Medical Association* 54: 256–59.

———. 1964a. "H.E.W. Conference on the Elimination of Hospital Discrimination." *Journal of the National Medical Association* 56: 446.

———. 1964b. "The Hospital Integration Story in Charlotte, North Carolina." *Journal of the National Medical Association* 56 (3): 226–29.

———. 1967. "Factors Influencing the Fate of the Negro Hospital." *Journal of the National Medical Association* 59: 217–19.

Cohen, Wilbur. 1966. "Memorandum to Henry Wills, the Attorney General, the Secretary of Labor and Director, Bureau of the Budget." White House Central Files. Austin, TX: Lyndon Baines Johnson Library.

Commission to End Health Care Disparities. 2010. "Five Year Summary Report." American Medical Association. *www.ama-assn.org/resources/doc/public-health/cehcd-five-year-summary.pdf*.

Committee on Intelligence Activities, Frank Church Chairman. Senate Report 94-755, "Intelligence Activities and the Rights of Americans." Edited by US Senate. Washington, DC: US Congress.

Conn, Robert. 1965. "Presbyterian Will Change Policy to Admit Negroes." *Charlotte Observer*, March 20, 1.

"Countries Compared by Health > Hospital beds > Per 1,000 people. International Statistics at NationMaster.com." 2015. World Development Indicators database. *www.nationmaster.com/country-info/stats/Health/Hospital-beds/Per-1,000-people*.

David Barton Smith Hospital Segregation Files. 2015. Blockson Collection. Philadelphia: Temple University Library.

Dallek, Robert. 1998. *Flawed Giant: Lyndon Johnson and His Times 1961–1973.* New York: Oxford University Press.

Dent, Albert. 1949. "Hospital Services and Facilities Available to Negroes in the United States." *Journal of Negro Education* 18 (3): 326–32.

Department of Health and Human Services. 2010. "Healthy People 2020." *www. healthypeople.gov/2020/default.aspx.*

Department of Health, Education and Welfare. 1966. Winder County Memorial Hospital Medical Facilities Compliance Report. David Barton Smith Hospital Segregation Files, Blockson Collection. Philadelphia: Temple University Library.

Dittmer, John. 2009. *The Good Doctors.* New York: Bloomsbury.

Douglas, Davidson M. 1994. "The Quest for Freedom in the Post-Brown South: Desegregation and White Self-Interest." *Chicago-Kent Law Review* 70: 689–755.

Duke University Medical School. "Trailblazer YouTube Video." *www.youtube. com/watch?v=gd-ih66t574.*

Eaton, Hubert A. 1984. *Every Man Should Try.* Wilmington, NC: Bonaparte.

Falk, Isadore, Margaret Klem, and Nathan Sinai. 1933. *The Incidence of Illness and the Receipt and Costs of Medical Care among Representative Families, Committee on the Cost of Medical Care* Report No. 27. Chicago: University of Chicago Press.

Falls, Arthur. 1988. Taped Interview with Arthur Falls by Walter Lear. Medical Committee for Human Rights Records. Rare Book and Manuscript Library. Philadelphia: University of Pennsylvania Library.

Feder, Judith. 1977. *Medicare: The Politics of Federal Hospital Insurance.* Lexington, MA: Lexington Books.

Friedson, Eliot. 1970. *Professional Dominance: The Social Structure of Medical Care.* New York: Atherton.

Galloway, Angela. 1999. "He Still Presses for Justice: A Compatriot of Dr. King's Spoke in Coatsville." *Philadelphia Inquirer,* February 1, B1.

Gardner, John. 1965a. "Memorandum to Executive Staff." In *OCR Historical Record: Title VI Implementation,* edited by Elaine Heffernan, 163–64. Austin, TX: Lyndon Baines Johnson Library.

———. 1965b. Telegram from John Gardner to John Holloman. Medical Committee for Human Rights Records. Rare Book and Manuscript Library. Philadelphia: University of Pennsylvania Library.

———. 2003. *Living, Leading and the American Dream.* San Francisco: Jossey-Bass.

Geiger, Jack. 1999. Letter from H. Jack Geiger to David B. Smith. David Barton Smith Hospital Segregation Files, Blockson Collection. Philadelphia: Temple University Library.

———. 2005. "The Unsteady March." *Perspectives in Biology and Medicine* 48 (1): 1–9.

———. 2013. Filmed Interview with Jack Geiger. In *Power to Heal Documentary*, edited by Barbara Berney. Astoria, NY: BLB Productions.

———. 2015. "Email Response to Manuscript." June 18. David Barton Smith Files, Blockson Collection. Temple University Library, Philadelphia.

Gluck, M. G., and V. Reno, eds. 2001. *Reflections on Implementing Medicare*. Washington, DC: National Academy of Social Insurance.

Golden, Harry. 1958. *Only in America*. Cleveland: World.

———. 1967. *The Best of Harry Golden*. Cleveland: World.

Greensboro Daily News. 1962. *Greensboro Daily News*, June 9, 1.

Haas, Jeffery. 2009. *The Assassination of Fred Hampton: How the FBI and the Chicago Police Murdered a Black Panther*. Chicago: Lawrence Hills Books.

Hansberry, Lorraine. 1970. *To Be Young Gifted and Black: Lorraine Hansberry in Her Own Words (Adapted by Robert Nemiroff)*. New York: Signet.

Harriman, Joy H. P. 2011. *Health Care in Mobile: An Oral History of the 1940's*. Mobile, AL: N.p.

Havighurst, Robert. 1964. *The Public Schools of Chicago: A Survey for the Board of Education of the City of Chicago*. Chicago: Board of Education of the City of Chicago.

Hereford, Sonnie Wellington, IV. 2007. "My Walk into History." *Notre Dame Magazine*, Spring 2007. *magazine.nd.edu/news/9874-my-walk-into-history*.

Hereford, Sonnie Wellington, III, and Jack D. Ellis. 2011. *Beside the Troubled Waters: A Black Doctor Remembers, Life, Medicine and Civil Rights in an Alabama Town*: Tuscaloosa: University of Alabama Press.

Hess, Arthur. 1991. "Recollections by Social Security Administration Officials' Knowledge and/or Involvement in Certain Stages of Early Implementation of the Medicare Program (Calendar Year 1966) and attached documents. David Barton Smith Hospital Segregation Files, Blockson Collection. Philadelphia: Temple University Library.

Hill-Rom. 2014. "Hill-Rom 2013 Annual Review." *//files.shareholder.com/downloads/HBI/3669866927x0x719785/61873375-6E89-441B-93D0-225F53270349/HR_CEO_letter_and_10k_011714b.pdf*.

Hirsch, Arnold R. 1983. *Making of the Second Ghetto: Race and Housing in Chicago 1940–1960*. Cambridge: Cambridge University Press.

Hoffman, Beatrix. 2012. *Health Care for Some: Rights and Rationing in the United States since 1930*. Chicago: University of Chicago Press.

Holloman, John. 1965a. Special Delivery Letter from Holloman to Gardner. Medical Committee for Human Rights Records. Rare Book and Manuscript Library. Philadelphia: University of Pennsylvania Library

———. 1965b. Telegram to Gardner from John Holloman. In Medical Committee for Human Rights Records. Rare Book and Manuscript Library. Philadelphia: University of Pennsylvania Library.

Holman, Mary. 1965. "Mary Holman Secretary of MCHR, Memorandum to John Parham, September 9." Medical Committee for Human Rights Records. Rare Book and Manuscript Library. Philadelphia: University of Pennsylvania Library.

"Infant Mortality Rates 1950–2010." n.d. Sandbox Networks publishing as Infoplease. *www.infoplease.com/ipa/A0779935.html.*

INS. 1955. "Six Women Best Males as Medical School Opens." Rpt. *New Orleans Times-Picayune,* January 2, 1966, 55.

Janssen, Kim. 2009. "62-Year-Old Kills 72-Year-Old over Stolen Nursing Home Dinner." *Chicago Sun Times,* December 16, 18.

Johnson, Carla K. 2009. "Deadly Mix: Mentally Ill in Nursing homes: Nationwide Problem Especially Bad Here." *Chicago Sun Times,* March 22, 1.

Johnson, Everett A. 1964. "The Civil Rights Act of 1964—What It Means for Hospitals." *Hospitals* 38 (November 16): 51–54.

Johnson, Lyndon Baines. 1963a. "Address before the Joint Session of Congress, November 27, 1963." Edited by Gerhard Peter and John T. Wooley. *American Presidency Project. www.presidency.ucsb.edu/ws/index.php?pid=25988.*

———. 1963b. "Johnson Conversation with Martin Luther King on Nov 25, 1963 (K6311.02)." Miller Center, University of Virginia. *millercenter.org/presidentialrecordings/lbj-k6311.02–22.*

———. 1963c. "Remarks at Gettysburg on Civil Right." May 30. Miller Center, University of Virginia. *millercenter.org/president/lbjohnson/speeches/speech-3380.*

———. 1966a. "Remarks at a Meeting with Medical and Hospital Leaders to Prepare for the Launching of Medicare, June 15, 1966." Edited by Gerhard Peters and John T. Wooley. *American Presidency Project. www.presidency.ucsb.edu/ws/index.php?pid=27650.*

———. 1966b. "Remarks to Members of the National Council of Senior Citizens, June, 3 1966." Edited by Gerhard Peters and John T. Wooley. *American Presidency Project. www.presidency.ucsb.edu/ws/index.php?pid=27630.*

———. 1966c. "Statement by the President on the Inauguration of the Medicare Program, June 30, 1966." Edited by Gerhard Peters and John T. Wooley. *American Presidency Project. www.presidency.ucsb.edu/ws/index.php?pid=27692.*

Johnson, Paul B. 1970. "Oral History Interview with Paul B. Johnson Jr. Interviewed by T. H. Baker, September 8, 1970." Miller Center, Courtesy of the LBJ Library, University of Virginia, Charlottesville. *web2.millercenter.org/lbj/oralhistory/johnson_paul_1970_0908.pdf.*

Jones, James H. 1981. *Bad Blood: The Tuskegee Syphilis Experiment.* New York: Free Press.

Journal of the National Medical Association. 1962. "Sixth Imhotep Conference Confident of Results from United Broad Effort." *Journal of the National Medical Association* 54 (4): 499, 502–3.

Joynt, K. E., E. J. Oray, and A. K. Jha. 2011. "Thirty-Day Readmission Rates for Medicare Beneficiaries by Race and Site of Care." *Journal of the American Medical Association* 305 (7): 675–81.

Kaiser Family Foundation. 2015a. "Federal Medical Assistance Percentage (FMAP) for Medicaid and Multiplier." Kaiser Family Foundation. *kff.org/medicaid/state-indicator/federal-matching-rate-and-multiplier*.

———. 2015b. "Status of State Action on Medicaid Decision." Kaiser Family Foundation. *kff.org/health-reform/state-indicator/state-activity-around-expanding-medicaid-under-the-affordable-care-act*.

Katzenbach, Nicholas D. 1968. "Interview I by Page E. Mulholland on, November 12, 1968." Miller Center, Courtesy of LBJ Library Oral History Collection. Charlottesville: University of Virginia. *web2.millercenter.org/lbj/oralhistory/katzenbach_nicholas_1968_1112.pdf*.

Kennedy, John F. 1962. "The President's Message." *Journal of the National Medical Association* 54 (4): 501.

———. 1964. "Special Message to Congress on Civil Rights and Job Opportunities, June 19, 1963." In *Public Papers of the Presidents of the United States: John F. Kennedy, 1963*, 492. Washington, DC: Government Printing Office.

King, Martin Luther. 1963. "I Have a Dream." American Rhetoric. *www.americanrhetoric.com/speeches/mlkihaveadream.htm*.

———. 1968. "I've Been to the Mountain Top." *www.americanrhetoric.com/speeches/mlkivebeentothemountaintop.htm*.

Kotz, Nick. 2005. *Judgment Days: Lyndon Baines Johnson, Martin Luther King Jr., and the Laws That Changed America*. New York: Houghton Mifflin.

Krieger, Nancy, David H. Rehkop, Jarvis T. Chen, Pamela D Waterman, Enrico Marcelli, and Malinda Kennedy. 2008. "The Fall and Rise of US Inequalities in Premature Mortality 1960–2002." *PLOS Medicine* 5 (2): 227–40.

Krock, Arthur. 1964. "A Court Ruling Extended to Pending Legislation." *New York Times*, March 5, 32.

Lasagna, Louis. 1965a. "Dr. Lasagna Reply to Dr. Marston's Letter." *Yale Journal of Biology and Medicine* 38 (August): 48.

———. 1965b. "The Mind and Morality of the Doctor: II. The Physician and the Macrocosm." *Yale Journal of Biology and Medicine* 37 (April): 362–63.

Lee, Philip. 1969. "Interview e. by David C. McComb. January 28." Miller Center, Courtesy of LBJ Library Oral History Collection. Charlottesville: University of Virginia. *web2.millercenter.org/lbj/oralhistory/lee_philip_1969_0128.pdf*.

Leflore, L. J. 1965a. "Letter to James Quigley." Non-partisan Voter's League Files, University of Southern Alabama Archives, Mobile, AL, March 24.

———.1965b. "Letter to James Quigley." Voter's League Files, University of Southern Alabama Archives, Mobile, AL, October 6.

Libassi, Peter. 1966. "Memo to Joseph Califano, Douglass Cater and Nicholas Katzenbach." Central White House Files, Lyndon Baines Johnson Library: Austin, TX, May 6.

Love, Spencie. 1996. *One Blood: The Death and Resurrection of Charles R. Drew.* Chapel Hill: University of North Carolina Press.

Lowenstein, Jeff Kelly. 2009. "Disparate Nursing Home Care." *Chicago Reporter,* July 1. *chicagoreporter.com/disparate-nursing-home-care.*

Ludwig, Jens, Lisa Sanbonmatsu, Lisa Gennetian, Emma Adam, Greg J. Dimcam, et al. 2011. "Neighborhoods, Obesity, and Diabetes—a Randomized Social Experiment." *New England Journal of Medicine* 365 (16): 1509–19.

Majerol, Melissa, Vann Newkirk, and Rachel Garfield. 2014. *The Uninsured: A Primer.* Washington, DC: Kaiser Commission on Medicaid and the Uninsured.

Marston, Robert Q. 1965. "Correspondence from the University of Mississippi Medical Center." *Yale Journal of Biology and Medicine* 38 (August): 48–49.

Martin, Ruby G. 1974. Oral History Interview with Ruby Martin by Thomas Harri Baker, Miller Center, Courtesy of LBJ Library Oral History Collection. Charlottesville: University of Virginia. *web2.millercenter.org/lbj/oralhistory/ martin_ruby_1969_0224.pdf.*

Maund, Alfred. 1952. *The Untouchables: The Meaning of Segregation in Hospitals.* Edited by Southern Conference Educational Fund Michael Davis Papers. New York: New York Academy of Medicine.

Medical World News. 1963. "Historic Decision on Segregation." *Medical World News,* November 23, 54–56.

Miller, Merle. 1980. *Lyndon: An Oral Biography.* New York: Putnam.

Mississippi Sovereignty Commission. 1964a. "Earle Johnson Memo to File on Coordinating Committee for Fundamental American Freedom January 14, 1964." Mississippi Department of Archives and History. *mdah.state.ms.us/ arrec/digital_archives/sovcom.*

———. 1964b. "The Socialist Omnibus Bill of 1963 (SCR ID #99-36-0-35-4-2-1-1-1 to SCRI ID # 99-36-0-4-3-1-13-1-1-1)." Mississippi Department of Archives and History. *mdah.state.ms.us/arrec/digital_archives/sovcom.*

Mobile Register. 1967. "Medicare Fight Won by Hospital." *Mobile Register,* February 23, 1.

Moore, Amanda. 2013. "Tracking Down Martin Luther King, Jr.'s Words on Health Care." Huffington Post. Last modified March 20, 2013. *www.huffingtonpost.com/amanda-moore/martin-luther-king-health-care_b_2506393.html.*

Mor, Vincent, Jackie Zinn, Joseph Angelelli, Joan M. Teno, and Susan C. Miller. 2004. "Driven to Tiers: Socioeconomic and Racial Disparities in Quality of Nursing Home Care." *Milbank Quarterly* 82 (2): 227–56.

Morris, John P. 1960. "The Denial of Staff Positions to Negro Physicians: A Violation of the Sherman Act." *Journal of the National Medical Association* 52 (3): 211–15.

Morris, Robert G. 1960. "The Problems in Securing Hospital Staff Appointments for Negro Physicians in Chicago." *Journal of the National Medical Association* 52 (3): 194–97.

Moses Cone Hospital Board. 1964. Minutes of the Executive Committee. Greensboro, NC: Moses Cone Hospital.

Moyers, Bill. 2003. "Foreword." In *Living, Leading the American Dream*, edited by Francesca Gardner, xiii–xvi. San Francisco: Jossey-Bass.

Myrdal, Gunnar. 1944. *The American Dilemma: The Negro Problem and Modern Democracy*. New York: Harper and Brothers.

NAACP Legal Defense Fund. 1965. *Report on Implementation of Title VI of the Civil Rights Act of 1964 in Regard to Hospital Discrimination: Recommendations for 1966*. Medical Committee for Human Rights Records. Rare Book and Manuscript Library. Philadelphia: University of Pennsylvania Library.

Nash, Robert M. 1966a. "Compliance of Hospitals and Health Agencies with Title VI of the Civil Rights Act." *American Journal of Public Health* 58 (2): 246–51.

———. 1966b. "Letter to L. S. Blades, III, Board Chairman Albermarley Hospital Inc." May 13. David Barton Smith Hospital Segregation Files, Blockson Collection. Philadelphia: Temple University Library.

National Center for Health Statistics. 1975. "Selected Operating and Financial Characteristics of Nursing Homes in the United States 1973–74." In *National Nursing Home Survey*. Washington, DC: National Center for Health Statistics.

———. 2014. *Health, United States, 2013*. Hyattsville, MD: National Center for Health Statistics.

"National Conference on Title VI—Civil Rights Act of 1964." 1965. *Journal of the National Medical Association* 57 (2): 163.

National Institutes of Health. 2013. "A Short History of the National Institutes of Health." *history.nih.gov/exhibits/history/index.html*.

Nelson, Alonda. 2011. *Body and Soul: The Black Panther Party and the Fight against Medical Discrimination*. Minneapolis: University of Minnesota Press.

Nesbit, Bonnie J. 1970. "Need Medics for Clinic." *Chicago Daily Defender*, August 12, 27.

Non-partisan Voters' League. 1965. "Willie James Myles Deposition." Non-partisan Voters League Files, Mobile: Southern Alabama University Library Archives.

Nordheimer, Jon. 2011. "Rev. Fred L. Shuttlesworth, an Elder Statesman for Civil Rights, Dies at 89." *New York Times*, October 6, A33. *www.nytimes.com/2011/10/06/us/rev-fred-l-shuttlesworth-civil-rights-leader-dies-at-89.html*.

North Carolina History Project. 2015. "Reginald Hawkins (1923–2007)." *www.northcarolinahistory.org/encyclopedia/300/entry*.

Oberlander, Jonathan, and Theodore R. Marmor. 2015. "The Road Not Taken: What Happened to Medicare for All?" In *Medicare and Medicaid at 50: America's Entitlement Programs in the Age of Affordable Care*, edited by

Alan B. Cohen, David C. Colby, Keith A. Wailoo, and Julian E. Zelizer, 55–74. New York: Oxford University Press.

OECD. 2014. "OECD Health Statistics 2014: How Does the United States Compare?" *www.oecd.org/unitedstates/Briefing-Note-UNITED-STATES-2014.pdf.*

OEHO. 1966. "Medical Facilities Compliance Report Winder County Memorial Hospital, North Carolina." David Barton Smith Hospital Segregation Files, Blockson Collection. Philadelphia: Temple University Library.

Oliver, K. 1985. "Illnesses of Bodies and Minds: Early Black Doctors Faced Both." *Miami Herald*, October 7, VC1, C3.

Olzak, Susan. 1992. *The Dynamics of Ethnic Competition and Conflict.* Stanford, CA: Stanford University Press.

Olzak, Susan, and Suzanne Shanahan. 2003. "Racial Policy and Racial Conflict in the Urban United States, 1869–1924." *Social Forces* 82 (2): 481–517.

Panetta, Leon, and Peter Gill. 1971. *Bring Us Together: The Nixon Team and the Civil Rights Retreat.* Philadelphia: Lippincott.

Parham, John. 1965. "Memorandum to Ruth Hurwitz." Medical Committee for Human Rights Records. Rare Book and Manuscript Library. Philadelphia: University of Pennsylvania Library.

Pear, Robert. 1996. "Federal Taxation Shows it Has 2 Faces." *New York Times*, October 8, A1, A23.

Plotz, Paul. 2000. Notes from Plotz Interview by P. Preston Reynolds. David Barton Smith Hospital Segregation Collection, Blockson Collection. Philadelphia: Temple University Library.

Poen, Monte M. 1979. *Harry S. Truman versus the Medical Lobby.* Columbia: University of Missouri Press.

Polikoff, Alexander. 2006. *Waiting for Gautreaux: A Story of Segregation, Housing and the Black Ghetto.* Evanston, IL: Northwestern University Press.

Pollack, Harold. 2015. "Medicare for All—If I Were Politically Possible—Would Necessarily Replicate the Defects of the Current System." *Journal of Health Politics, Policy and Law* 40 (4): 921–29.

Poussaint, Alvin. 1965. "Letter from Poussaint to Representatives Burton, Mathias, Powell, and Kastenmeier and Senators Javits and Kennedy." Medical Committee for Human Rights Records, HEW Correspondence Files. Rare Book and Manuscript Library. Philadelphia: University of Pennsylvania Library.

Quadagno, Jill. 1994. *The Color of Welfare: How Racism Undermined the War on Poverty.* Oxford: Oxford University Press.

Quigley, James. 1961. "Memorandum to Harris Wofford." Harris Wofford Papers. Boston: John F. Kennedy Library.

Quinn, Janis. 2005. *Promises Kept: The University of Mississippi Medical Center.* Jackson: University Press of Mississippi.

Raines, Howell. 2015. "The Dream World of the Southern Republicans." *New York Times*, July 10. *www.nytimes.com/2015/07/12/opinion/sunday/will-demographics-transform-southern-politics.html*.

Reagan, Ronald. 1980. "Neshoba County Fair Speech." *www.onlinemadison.com/ftp/reagan/reaganneshoba.mp3*.

Reid, T. R. 2010. *The Healing of America: The Global Quest for Better, Cheaper and Fairer Health Care*. New York: Penguin.

Reinhardt, Uwe E. 2015. "Medicare Innovations in the War over the Keys to the US Treasury." In *Medicare and Medicaid at 50: America's Entitlement Programs in the Age of Affordable Care*, edited by Alan B. Cohen, David C. Colby, Keith A. Wailoo, and Julian E. Zelizer, 169–89. New York: Oxford University Press.

Reynolds, P. Preston. 1997. "The Federal Government's Use of Title VI and Medicare to Racially Integrate Hospitals in the United States 1963–1967." *American Journal of Public Health* 87 (11): 1851–57.

———. 2004. "Professional and Hospital Discrimination and the US Court of Appeals Fourth Circuit 1956–1967." *American Journal of Public Health* 94: 710–20.

Rice, Jon F. 1998. "Black Radicalism on Chicago's West Side: A History of the Illinois Black Panther Party." PhD diss., Northern Illinois University.

Richardson, Michael B. 2005. "'Not Gradually . . . but Now': Reginald Hawkins, Black Leadership and Desegregation in Charlotte, North Carolina." *North Carolina Historical Review* 82 (3): 347–79.

Rose, Marilyn. 1997. Memo to David Smith. David Barton Smith Hospital Segregation Collection, Blockson Collection. Philadelphia: Temple University Library.

Rosenbaum, Sara. 2013. *Principles to Consider for the Implementation of a Community Health Needs Assessment Process*. Washington, DC: George Washington University.

Roth, Charles. 1964. "Note from Charles Roth to Harold Bettis." Greensboro, NC: Moses Cone Hospital Historical Collection.

Rucker, Philip. 2009. "Sen. DeMint of S.C. Is Voice of Opposition to Health Care Reform." *Washington Post*, July 28. *www.washingtonpost.com/wp-dyn/content/article/2009/07/27/AR2009072703066.html*.

Sandburg, Carl. 1919. *The Chicago Race Riots July 1919*. New York: Harcourt Brace.

Schiller, Emily Rose. 2008. "'To Give Medicine Back to the People': Community Health Activism of the Panther Party." Undergraduate honors thesis, Professor Regina Morantz-Sanchez, advisor, University of Michigan.

Schlesinger, Mark. 2015. "Medicare and the Social Transformations of American Elders." In *Medicare and Medicaid at 50: America's Entitlement Programs in the Age of Affordable Care*, edited by Alan B. Cohen, David C. Colby, Keith A. Wailoo, and Julian E. Zelizer, 119–44. New York: Cambridge University Press.

Seidman, Larry. 2015. "The Affordable Care Act versus Medicare for All." *Journal of Health Politics, Policy and Law* 40 (4): 909–19.

Shem, Samuel. 1995. *The House of God*. New York: Dell.

Shervington, Walter W. 2000. "Discrimination among Major Health Plans Plague Nation's Minority Physicians and Patients." *Journal of the National Medical Association* 92 (3): 103–4.

Shuttlesworth, Fred. 2004. "Fred Shuttlesworth Speaks in Philadelphia." *Philadelphia Inquirer*. B1.

Simpson, Dick. 2001. *Rogues, Rebels and Rubber Stamps: The Politics of the Chicago City Council from 1863 to the Present*. Chicago: Westview.

Sisti, Dominic A., Andrea G. Segal, and Ezekiel J. Emanuel. 2015. "Improving Long-Term Psychiatric Care: Bring Back the Asylum." *JAMA* 313 (3): 243–44.

Smith, David B. 1998. "The Racial Segregation of Hospital Care Revisited: Medicare Discharge Patterns and Their Implications." *American Journal of Public Health* 88 (3): 461–63.

———. 1999. *Health Care Divided: Race and Healing a Nation*. Ann Arbor: University of Michigan Press.

———. 2003. *Reinventing Care: Assisted Living in New York City*. Nashville: Vanderbilt University Press.

———. 2005. "The Politics of Disparities: Desegregating the Hospitals in Jackson, Mississippi." *Milbank Quarterly* 83 (5): 247–69.

———. 2009. *Forensic Case Files*. Singapore: World Scientific.

———. 2014. "Minorities, Immigrants and Health Care Policy: Disparities and Solutions." In *Guide to U.S. Health and Health Care Policy*, edited by Thomas Oliver, 293–306. New York: DWJ Books.

———. 2015a. "Civil Rights and Medicare: Historical Convergence and Continuing Legacy." In *Medicare and Medicaid at 50: America's Entitlement Programs in the Age of Affordable Care*, edited by Alan B. Cohen, David C. Colby, Keith A. Wailoo, and Julian E. Zelizer, 22–38. New York: Oxford University Press.

———. 2015b. "The 'Golden Rules' for Eliminating Disparities: Title VI, Medicare and the Implementation of the Affordable Care Act." *Health Matrix: Journal of Law and Medicine* 25: 33–60.

Smith, David Barton, Zhanlian Feng, Mary L. Fennell, Jacqueline S. Zinn, and Vincent Mor. 2007. "Separate and Unequal: Racial Segregation and Disparities in Quality across U.S. Nursing Homes." *Health Affairs* 26 (5): 1448–58.

"Racial Disparities in Access to Long-Term Care: The Illusive Pursuit of Equity." *Journal of Health Politics, Policy and Law* 33 (5): 861–81.

Squires, David A. 2012 "The U.S. Health System in Perspective: A Comparison of Twelve Industrialized Nations." *Issues in International Health Policy*. New York: Commonwealth Fund. Pub. 1595. Vol. 10, May. *www.commonwealthfund. org/~/media/Files/Publications/Issue%20Brief/2012/May/1595_Squires_ explaining_high_hlt_care_spending_intl_brief.pdf*.

Starr, Paul. 1982. *The Social Transformation of American Medicine*. New York: Basic Books.

———. 2015. "Built to Last? Policy Retrenchment and Regret in Medicare, Medicaid and the Affordable Care Act. In *Medicare and Medicaid at 50: America's Entitlement Programs in the Age of Affordable Care*, edited by Alan B. Cohen, David C. Colby, Keith A. Wailoo, and Julian E. Zelizer, 321–31. New York: Oxford University Press.

Steif, William. 1967. "The New Look in Civil Rights Enforcement." *Southern Education Report* 3 (2): 2–7.

Stone, Deborah. 1993. "The Struggle for the Soul of Health Insurance." *Journal of Health Politics, Policy and Law* 18 (2): 287–318.

Stovel, Katherine. 2001. "Local Sequential Patterns: The Structure of Lynching in the Deep South, 1882–1930." *Social Forces* 79 (3): 843–80.

Substance Abuse and Mental Health Services Administration. 2008. *Funding and Characteristics of State Mental Health Agencies 2007*. Rockville, MD: Substance Abuse and Mental Health Services Administration, Department of Health and Human Services (SAMHSA, HHS).

Taylor, G. Flint, and Ben H. Elson. 2009. "The Assassination of Fred Hampton: 40 Years Later." *Police Misconduct and Civil Rights Law Report* 9 (12): 1–12. *peopleslawoffice.com/wp-content/uploads/2012/02/Nov.Dec_.2009.PMCRLR. Galleys.pdf*.

Teitelbaum, Joel, Lara Cartwright-Smith, and Sara Rosenbaum. 2012. "Translating Rights into Access: Language Access and the Affordable Care Act." *American Journal of Law and Medicine* 38 (2–3): 348–73.

"Third Meeting of the AMA-NMA Representatives." 1964. *Journal of the National Medical Association* 56 (1): 103–4.

Thomas, Karen Kruse. 2011. *Deluxe Jim Crow: Civil Rights and American Health Policy 1935–1954*. Athens: University of Georgia Press.

Thompson, Frank J. 2015. "Medicaid Rising: The Perils and Potential of Federalism." In *Medicare and Medicaid at 50: America's Entitlement Programs in the Age of Affordable Care*, edited by Alan B. Cohen, David C. Colby, Keith A. Wailoo, and Julian E. Zelizer, 192–229. New York: Oxford University Press.

Tidwell, Mike. 2000. "The Quiet Revolution." *American Legacy* 6 (2): 25–32.

"Title VI and Hospitals." 1966. *Journal of the National Medical Association* 58 (3): 212–13.

Torrey, E. Fuller, Doris A. Fuller, Jeffrey Geller, Carla Jacobs, and Kristina Ragosta. 2012. *No Room at the Inn: Trends and Consequences of Closing Public Psychiatric Hospitals*. Washington, DC: Treatment Advocacy Center. *ww1.prweb.com/prfiles/2012/07/18/9703740/No_Room_at_the_Inn-2012. pdf*.

Trott, Bill. 2015. "U.S. Issues New Rule to Promote Racial Integration in Housing." Last modified July 8, 2015. *www.reuters.com/article/2015/07/08/ us-usa-housing-idUSKCN0PI1HZ20150708*.

Undergrove, Mark K. 2014. "What 'Selma' Gets Wrong: LBJ and MLK Were Close Partners in Reform." *Politico Magazine*, December 22. *www.politico.com/magazine/story/2014/12/what-selma-gets-wrong-113743_full.html*.

United States Commission on Civil Rights. 1966. *Title VI . . . One Year After: A Survey of Desegregation of Health and Welfare Services in the South.* Washington, DC: US Government Printing Office.

———. 1970. *HEW and Title VI.* Washington, DC: US Government and Printing Office.

US Bureau of the Census. 1960. *Decennial Census.* Washington, DC.

———. 2010. *American Community Survey.* Washington, DC: US Bureau of the Census.

———. 2012. *Statistical Abstract of the United States: 2012.* Washington, DC: US Department of Commerce. *www.census.gov/library/publications/time-series/statistical_abstracts.html*.

US Department of Health and Human Services. 1991. *Healthy People 2000: National Health Promotion and Disease Objectives.* Washington, DC: Department of Health and Human Services.

———. 2000. *Healthy People 2010: Understanding and Improving Health.* 2nd ed. 2 vols. Washington, DC: US Government Printing Office.

Wallace, George. 1963. "1963 Inaugural Address." *digital.archives.alabama.gov/cdm/singleitem/collection/voices/id/2952/rec/5*.

Watson, Sydney. 2012. "Section 1557 of the Affordable Care Act: Civil Rights, Health Care Reform, Race and Equity." *Howard Law Journal* 55 (Spring): 855–86.

Weare, Walter B. 1993. *Black Business in the New South: A Social History of the NC Mutual Life Insurance Company.* Durham, NC: Duke University Press.

Wesley, Nathaniel. 2010. *Black Hospitals in America: History, Contributions and Demise.* Tallahassee, FL: NRW.

Whalen, Charles, and Barbara Whalen. 1985. *The Longest Debate: A Legislative History of the 1964 Civil Rights Act.* Edited by US Senate. Washington, DC: Seven Locks Press.

White House. 1966. *President Lyndon B. Johnson Daily Diary.* Edited by White House. Austin, TX: Lyndon Baines Johnson Library.

Wilkerson, Isabel. 2010. *The Warmth of Other Suns: The Epic Story of America's Great Migration.* New York: Random House.

Wilkins, Roy, and Arnold Aronson. 1961. *Proposal for Executive Action to End Federally Supported Segregation and Other Forms of Discrimination.* White House Central Files. Boston: John F. Kennedy Library.

Williams, Jeanette. 1970. "Panthers Defend Clinic." *Chicago Daily Defender*, May 7, 4.

Wire Service. 1965. "Coalition of Liberal Groups Today Accused the HEW Department of Failing to Implement Federal Desegregation Policy in the Medical Field." Medical Committee for Human Rights Records, Rare Book and Manuscript Library. Philadelphia: University of Pennsylvania Library, December 16.

Woods, Randall. 2006. *LBJ: Architect of American Ambition*. New York: Free Press.

Yerkes, H. M. 1966. "Letter to Senators Herman E. Talmadge and Richard B. Russell." Robert Ball Correspondence Files, Social Security Administration Archives. Baltimore: Social Security Administration.

Zelizer, Julian E. 2015. "The Contentious Origins of Medicare and Medicaid." In *Medicare and Medicaid at 50: America's Entitlement Programs in the Age of Affordable Care*, edited by Alan B. Cohen, David C. Colby, Keith A. Wailoo, and Julian E. Zelizer, 3–20. New York: Oxford University Press.

Zheng, Haochi, and Chao Zhou. 2009. "The Impact of Civil Rights Acts and Hospital Integration on Black-White Differences in Mortality: A Case Study of Motor Vehicle Accident Death Rates." Working Paper, Department of Economics, Minneapolis: University of Minnesota, 1–34. *artsandscience. usask.ca/economics/research/pdf/ChaoZhouBUMarch2509.pdf*.

Index

Abernathy, Ralph, 164
abortions, 166
Affordable Care Act (2010)
    community health needs assessment
        and, 181, 197–98
    federally qualified community health
        centers and, 201n2
    health equality and, 197–98
    Medicaid and, 193, 205n2
    resistance to, 3, 205–6n9
Afro-American Patrolman's League, 166
Agent X, 34
Alamance General Hospital (Burlington,
    North Carolina), 7
Albemarle Hospital in Elizabeth City,
    North Carolina, 125–26
Alexander, Fred, 47
Alexander, Kelly, 44, 47
"all deliberate speed" approach, 86, 93,
    107–8, 116
Alpha Kappa Alpha (black sorority), 30
American Civil Liberties Union, 176
American College of Surgeons (ACS), 20
American Dilemma, The (Myrdal), 2, 194
American exceptionalism, 2
American Hospital Association (AHA),
    52–53, 80, 83, 86, 197
American Medical Association (AMA)
    current policies of, 197
    Drew and, 7
    Imhotep conferences and, 52–53
    Medicare and, 85–86, 136–37
    Simkins case and, 80

"socialism" and, 28–29, 72
    on voluntary way, 25
    volunteer physicians in Vietnam and,
        137
*American Medical Association v. United
    States* (1943), 72
American Red Cross, 6–7
American Veterans Committee (AVC),
    15, 114
Anderson, Alan B., 89, 90
Anderson, Marion, 43
anti-Vietnam War activists, 33
Armstrong, Brenda, 9
Armstrong, Wiley T., 9, 56–57
Arnstein, Sherry, 57, 66, 108
Associated Negro Press, 49
Atlanta, Georgia, 80, 127
"Atlanta Compromise" (1895), 204n12
Atlantic City, New Jersey, 85
Avery, Maltheus, 7–8, 16

Ball, Robert, 106, 107, 110, 119–20, 139,
    141–44
Baptist Hospital (Jackson, Mississippi),
    146
Battle, Clinton, 32, 35, 36
Bell, Derrick, 108
Bell, Ezekiel, 39
Bernstein, Leon, 139
Berry, Leonidas, 159
Bettis, Harold, 81
Birmingham, Alabama, 76, 158–59
black churches, 52

227

riots (1968) in, 161, 172
school debacle in, 88–94, 103, 106
Chicago Black Panthers, 177–78, 192
Chicago Board of Education, 88–94
Chicago Commission on Human
Relations, 73–74
Chicago Daily Defender (newspaper),
14, 159, 162, 165
Chicago Daily News (newspaper), 11
Chicago Freedom Movement (CFM),
160–61, 175–77
Chicago Housing Authority (CHA),
176
Chicago School Board, 159
Chicago Urban League, 88
Childers, Bobby, 123, 171
Cicero, Illinois, 13–14
Civil Rights Act (1964)
Chicago school debacle and, 88–94,
103, 106
legislative history of, 76–83
residential segregation and, 176–77
See also Title VI compliance in
Medicare
Civil Rights Leadership Council, 65
Civil Rights Memorial (Montgomery,
Alabama), 146
civil rights movement
change effected by, 178–92
class divisions in, 47–48
legacy of, 175–78
role of presidential decisions in,
63–65
students and, 48
Title VI compliance in Medicare
and, 118–19
See also black health professionals;
specific civil rights activists
Clark, Jim, 138, 158–59
Cobb, W. Montague
on black cadavers and research, 23
as civil rights activist, 48–53, 61–62,
73, 83, 169
Cornely and, 168
Drew and, 7

Hawkins and, 43–44
Medicare and, 85–86
Cohen, Wilbur
Chicago school debacle and, 91
Title VI compliance in Medicare and,
106–7, 109, 119, 138–39, 140, 144,
170, 172
COINTELPRO (Counter Intelligence
Program), 32–33, 162–64, 174
College of Medical Evangelist (Loma
Linda, California; now Loma Linda
University), 30
Commission to End Health Care
Disparities, 197
Committee to End Discrimination in
Chicago's Medical Institutions, 17,
74, 89, 159, 166
community health needs assessment,
181, 197
Community Service Committee (CSC),
39, 40
community-based services, 190
"Compulsory Health Insurance—
Political Medicine—Is Bad Medicine
for America!" (pamphlet), 28
Congress of Racial Equality (CORE),
29, 48
Connor, Bull, 76, 158–59
Consolidated Budget Reconciliation Act
(COBRA, 1986), 209n3
contact stations, 120
Cook County Hospital (Chicago,
Illinois), 16–17, 20, 23, 24, 74, 159
Cook County Physicians Association,
165
Coordinating Committee for
Fundamental American Freedom,
77–78, 82, 88, 94
Coordinating Council of Community
Organizations (CCCO), 88–94, 158,
160
Cornely, Paul, 24, 25–26, 168
Courts, Gus, 35, 36
Cowsert, Jean, 135–36, 146–47, 149–58
critical race theory, 108

Culturally and Linguistically
Appropriate Services (CLAS)
Standards, 182–83
Cunningham, Marion, 118

Daly, Richard, 73–74, 91–92, 159, 161,
166
Davis, Joseph Emory, 202n2
De La Beckwith, Byron, 33
death rates, 22, 180
deinstitutionalization, 189–90
Delisle, Eric, 208n1
Department of Health, Education and
Welfare (HEW)
centralization of civil rights
enforcement in, 168–73
Chicago school debacle and, 88–94,
103, 106
Gardner as secretary of, 102–4
image of, 103–4
Imhotep conferences and, 52
team at, 105–10
Wofford and, 65–66
See also Office of Equal Health
Opportunity (OEHO); Public
Health Service (PHS); Title VI
compliance in Medicare
Department of Housing and Urban
Development (HUD), 177
Department of Justice (DOJ), 93, 117
desegregation
contact stations and, 120
golf courses and, 59–60
medical societies and, 44, 55–56
military and federal agencies and, 18,
44, 65
nursing homes and, 187–89, 190–92,
191 (fig.)
public accommodations and, 32,
44–45
schools and, 31–32, 41–43, 88–94,
132, 182
See also hospital segregation and
desegregation
"deserving poor," 19

Detroit Receiving Hospital (Detroit,
Michigan), 53–54
Diagnostic Related Group (DRG)
payments, 210n9
Dirksen, Everett, 90–91, 160
"disparate impact" and "disparate
treatment," 196
Dixiecrats, 174
Doctor, The (Fildes), 28
*Dorothy Gautreaux v. Chicago Housing
Authority*, 176
Douglas, Paul, 160
Drake, Harold Fanning, 38
Drew, Charles, 6–7, 48, 53, 54
Du Bois, W. E. B., 54
Duke University Medical Center
(Durham, North Carolina), 7–8, 16
Duke University Medical School
(Durham, North Carolina), 67
duty to care, 19, 21–23, 180

Eastland, Jim, 78
Eaton, Hubert, 25, 26, 56–57, 118, 168
Edwards, Jack, 208n6
elections (1966), 160, 169
Elementary and Secondary Education
Act (1965), 88–94, 101–2, 158
Ellis, Jack, 203n4
Emergency Medical Treatment and
Active Labor Act (EMTALA, 1986),
181
Ervin, Sam, 126
Evers, Medgar, 31, 33, 36, 77, 114

Fair Housing Act (1968), 136
Falls, Arthur, 73
Federal Bureau of Investigation (FBI),
32–33, 162–64, 174
Federally Qualified Neighborhood
Health Centers, 177
fee-for-service medical practice, 28–29
Ferebee, Dorothy, 30
Field of Dreams (film), 113
Fildes, Samuel Luke, 28
Flood, Daniel, 171

Title VI compliance in Medicare and, 83, 86–88, 116, 133–40, 144
Vietnam War and, 169
War on Poverty and, 88
Johnson, Paul, 149
Johnson, T. V., 36
Johnson C. Smith College, 43
Johnson Library, 63
Joint Commission for Accreditation of Healthcare Organizations (JCAHO), 180
Joint Commission on Accreditation of Hospitals, 20
Journal of the National Medical Association (journal), 49, 50, 52, 73

Kaplan, Allen, 118
Kastenmeier, Robert, 95–96
Kate B. Reynolds Memorial Hospital (Winston-Salem, North Carolina), 26
Katz, Lawrence F., 177
Katzenbach, Nicholas
  Chicago school debacle and, 91, 93
  federal civil rights responsibilities and, 98
  Title VI compliance in Medicare and, 87, 104, 132, 140
Keeler, Garrison, 158
Kennedy, John F.
  black vote and, 64–65
  Civil Rights Bill and, 76–78
  election of, 182
  executive inaction of, 65–66
  Imhotep Conference and, 61–62
  King and, 63–64
  medical school hospitals and, 66–70
  Simkins case and, 74–76
Kennedy, Robert, 46, 64, 75
Kennedy, Ted, 95–96
Kenney, John A., Sr., 49
Keppel, Francis, 90, 91, 93
King, Coretta, 64
King, Martin Luther
  assassination of, 161, 172
  Chicago and, 89, 146, 158–59, 160, 161

Hawkins and, 167
Howard and, 35–36
in Huntsville, 39
"I have a dream" speech by, 41–42
incarceration of, 63–64
on injustice in healthcare, 117
Johnson and, 78
Klinger, Alfred, 165
Knights and Daughters of Tabor, 30, 32
Ku Klux Klan (KKK), 42

L. Richardson Hospital (Greensboro, North Carolina), 60–61, 168
Lasagna, Louis, 147–48
Lau v. Nichols (1973), 182–83
Lee, George, 35, 36, 140
Lee, Philip, 119
Leflore, J. L., 154, 157
Libassi, Peter
  Martin and, 92
  role at HEW of, 105–9
  Title VI compliance in Medicare and, 114, 116, 132, 135, 144, 172
life expectancy, 1
Lin, Maya, 146
Lincoln Hospital (Durham, North Carolina), 7–8, 25, 54–55, 168–69, 204n20
Lincoln Memorial (Washington, DC), 41–42
Lippmann, Walter, 12, 30
local medical societies
  Black Panther Clinic and, 165
  Medicare and, 136
  segregation and desegregation in, 37–38, 44, 48–49, 55–56
  "socialism" and, 28, 72
Look (magazine), 14
Los Angeles, California
  urban riots (1965) in, 87, 101–2
  urban riots (1992) in, 177
Louisiana Red Cross Blood Bank, 125
Lying-in Hospital (Chicago, Illinois), 15

Magnolia Life Insurance Company, 30–31